Critical Thinking
In Nursing

A PRACTICAL
APPROACH

Critical Thinking In Nursing

A PRACTICAL APPROACH

ROSALINDA ALFARO-LeFEVRE, MSN, RN

President, Teaching Smart/Learning Easy
Malvern, Pennsylvania, and
West Chester, Pennsylvania

W.B. SAUNDERS COMPANY
A Division of Harcourt Brace & Company
PHILADELPHIA LONDON TORONTO
MONTREAL SYDNEY TOKYO

W.B. SAUNDERS COMPANY
A Division of Harcourt Brace & Company

The Curtis Center
Independence Square West
Philadelphia, Pennsylvania 19106

Library of Congress Cataloging-in-Publication Data

Alfaro-LeFevre, Rosalinda.
    Critical thinking in nursing: a practical approach / Rosalinda
Alfaro-LeFevre.

        p.   cm.

    Includes bibliographical references.

    ISBN 0–7216–5897–0

    1. Nursing.   2. Critical thinking.   I. Title.
    [DNLM: 1. Decision Making.   2. Nursing Process.   WY 100 A385c
    1995]
    RT86.A34   1995   610.73—dc20
    DNLM/DLC   94-25233

Critical Thinking in Nursing
A Practical Approach   ISBN 0–7216–5897–0

Printed in the United States of America.

Last digit is the print number: 9   8   7   6   5   4   3   2

Dedication

In Memory of Susie Giedgowd
July 22, 1953–June 24, 1994

Her courage, sense of humor, and commitment to her children—Tommy, Michael, and Sara—always prevailed, even when faced with leukemia.

Life's Precious Secret

She told me that she was the happiest person on earth and fully contented. How did this happen, and what were the causes?

She told me that the secrets were to always think of the other person first.

To enjoy each day through the endless small daily routines that in retrospect are so important.

To love your children by giving them the time and patience that is dearly needed when growing up in today's world.

And finally to be able to teach others these precious secrets so that they may also be able to reap the rewards.

Not until the end of her earthly life did I fully understand the enormous love and power that was generated by practicing these secrets each day.

She had it all figured out, the true meaning of love. I saw this love come back to her in much larger amounts than what she gave out.

She can never be replaced, just like the true meaning of love.

TOM GIEDGOWD

Consultants/Reviewers

I'm most grateful to the following individuals. Without their timely and insightful reviews and suggestions, this book wouldn't have been possible.

- **DORIS M. ALFARO, SRN (Great Britain)**   Retired, West Chester, Pennsylvania
- **LEDJIE BALLARD, MSN, CRNA**   Manager, Anesthesia Services, Group Health Cooperative, East Side Hospital, Seattle, Washington
- **MARGARET E. BRIODY, MSN, RN**   Associate Professor of Nursing, University of Rochester, Rochester, New York
- **KATHY BROGAN, MSN, MSHEd, RN**   Director of Education and Research, Presbyterian Hospital, Philadelphia, Pennsylvania
- **KATHRYN DEXHEIMER, RN, MSN**   Visiting Nurse Association, Kansas City, Missouri
- **NANCY M. FLYNN, RNC, MSN**   Clinical Educator, Bryn Mawr Hospital, Bryn Mawr, Pennsylvania
- **PAULINE M. GREEN PhD, RN**   Assistant Professor, Howard University, College of Nursing, Washington, DC
- **JOAN M. JENKS, PhD, RN**   Director, Baccalaureate Nursing Division, Thomas Jefferson University, Philadelphia, Pennsylvania
- **SHARON E. JOHNSON, MSN, RNC**   Nurse Manager, Cooper Hospital/University Medical Center, Camden, New Jersey
- **SUSAN S. JOHNSON, RN, MSN**   Guilford Technical Community College, Jamestown, North Carolina
- **DONNA M. KAUFFMAN, RN, MS**   Associate Professor, School of Nursing, Purdue University, West Lafayette, Indiana
- **ANN E. KELLY, MSN, RNCS**   Clinical Nurse Specialist, Health Care For Homeless Veterans, San Diego Veteran Affairs Medical Center, San Diego, California
- **HEIDI LAIRD MLA, BA, Cert. El. Ed.**   Malvern, Pennsylvania
- **LAVON LOCKWOOD, MSN, RN**   Assistant Professor, San Antonio Community College, San Antonio, Texas

▶ **CAROL R. MATZ, MSN, RN**   Assistant Professor, Department of Nursing, West Chester University, West Chester, Pennsylvania

▶ **MARYCAROL McGOVERN, PhD, RN**   Assistant Professor, College of Nursing, Villanova University, Villanova, Pennsylvania

▶ **KATHLEEN A. McMULLEN, PhD (c), RN**   Assistant Professor, Nursing Department, Holy Family College, Philadelphia, Pennsylvania

▶ **TERRI PATTERSON, CRRN, MSN**   Nursing Consultation Services, Norristown, Pennsylvania

▶ **LINDA PICKLESIMER, MSN, RN**   Instructor, Nursing Department, Greenville Technical College, Greenville, South Carolina

▶ **REBECCA RFSH, MEd**   Coordinator of Licensing and Accrediting, Director, Cognitive Remediation/Special Education, Mediplex Rehabilitation Center, Camden, New Jersey

▶ **CONSTANCE SECHRIST, RN**   Philadelphia, Pennsylvania

▶ **PAIGE M. STARR, RN**   New Graduate of: Massasoit Community College, Brockton, Massachusetts

▶ **SUSANNE NANCY SUCHI, MSN, RN**   Instructor/Lead Teacher, Department of Nursing, Henry Ford Community College, Dearborn, Michigan

▶ **CAROL TAYLOR, Ph.D. Candidate, MSN**   Clinical Ethicist and Assistant Professor, Nursing, Georgetown University, Washington, DC

▶ **THERESA M. VALIGA, EdD, RN**   Professor and Program Director, Graduate Nursing Program, Villanova University, Villanova, Pennsylvania

▶ **DENISE D. WILSON, PhD, RN**   Dean of Academic Affairs, Mennonite College of Nursing, Bloomington, Illinois

▶ **MARGARET ZAZO, MSN, MS, RN**   Instructor, Brandywine School of Nursing, Coatesville, Pennsylvania

Preface

What's Practical About This Approach?

Based on the premise that most of you already know a lot about how to think well, this book helps you *connect* with what you already know, and build on that knowledge. Recognizing you developed your own style of thinking long before now, it encourages you to identify strategies to think critically in your *own* way. With the help of examples, stories, illustrations, and practice exercises, you'll *use* critical thinking as you're learning about critical thinking. Chapters 1 and 2 focus on developing *general attitudes* of critical thinkers and learning *general critical thinking strategies*. Once you have this foundation, you can then master Chapters 3, 4, and 5 content—critical thinking in nursing—more readily.

More Specifically:

- **Chapter 1 (Overview: What Is Critical Thinking, and Why Is It Important?)** defines critical thinking, explains why we need to learn more about it, and emphasizes the importance of developing attitudes of critical thinkers. Although it provides an applied definition for critical thinking in nursing and uses some nursing examples, the main focus is on using critical thinking in our everyday lives.
- **Chapter 2 (How to Think Critically)** focuses on identifying ways to improve thinking. It explains *what* factors influence your ability to think well, *why* these factors are so influential, and *how* to develop strategies to use this knowledge to your advantage. Skills essential to critical thinking (e.g., identifying assumptions) are introduced, together with nursing examples of how the skills are used.
- **Chapters 3 and 4 (Critical Thinking in Nursing: An Overview; and Critical Thinking in Nursing: Beyond Clinical Judgment)** build on Chapter 1 and 2 content, addressing *critical thinking common to nurses*. Chapter 3 presents an overview of critical thinking in nursing, and goes on to address how to develop clinical judgment. Chapter 4 continues the discussion in Chapter 3, focusing on how to use critical thinking to make ethical decisions, apply nursing research, teach others and ourselves, and take tests.

- **Chapter 5 (Practicing Critical Thinking Skills)** provides opportunities to practice the skills first introduced in Chapter 2 in clinical nursing situations. Each skill is presented in the following format: name of the skill, definition of the skill, why the skill promotes critical thinking, how to accomplish the skill, and practice exercises for using the skill.

Design Elements and Writing Style

Great pains have been taken to include design elements that motivate you to want to read and allow you to use your own way of mastering content (see page xii, *The Best Way to Read This Book*). The writing style is informal, interactive, and designed to make you feel like "you're right there" talking with the author or having to make clinical decisions about the situations presented.

Instructors' Guide Available

To free faculty to direct creative energies toward *refining and improving* teaching strategies, rather than starting from scratch, an instructor's guide is available. This guide provides such things as:

- Innovative, practical teaching strategies
- Methods of outcome measurement, including how to use this book at a beginning level and how to revisit content as students progress to more advanced levels
- Bibliographic citations with synopses of helpful critical thinking references

A Word About "Patient/Client," The Scenarios, and "He/She"

Whenever possible, a fictitious name, or "someone," "person," "consumer," or "individual" is used (instead of "patient" or "client") to help us keep in mind that each patient or client is an *individual* who has unique needs, values, perceptions, and motivations. Many of the scenarios are situations that really happened. However, the names of the individuals and some of the facts have been altered to provide anonymity. *He* and *she* are used interchangeably to avoid the awkwardness of using "he or she" all the time.

Please Tell Us What You Think

We want to hear your struggles and concerns. Whether you're a student or faculty member, if you're having a problem with something, it's likely others are too. Your problems are our opportunities to learn, improve, and help others with the same concerns. Please let us know what you think. Address comments to Thomas Eoyang, Vice President and Editor-in-Chief, Nursing Books, W.B. Saunders Company, The Curtis Center, Independence Square West, Philadelphia, PA 19106.

ROSALINDA ALFARO-LEFEVRE

The Best Way to Read This Book

The Best Way to Read This Book Is However You *Choose* to Read It

1. For those of you who like the traditional approach, read it from beginning to end. You'll enjoy the narrative, logical approach, and numerous scenarios and examples designed to help you understand and *remember* content.
2. For those of you who like to use your own unique approach—for example, the *back to front* approach (read summaries before text), the *skip around to the stuff that looks interesting* approach, or the *read the stuff that will be on the test first* approach—here are some of the features that help you focus on what's most important.

Preceding Each Chapter

- **This Chapter At a Glance:** Allows you to scan major headings.
- **Why Read This Chapter?** Presents a pre-test and objectives to help you decide how to focus your thinking about content, and where to spend most of your time.
- **Abstract:** Gives the big picture of what the chapter is all about.

Following Each Chapter

- **Key Points:** Provide a detailed summary of the most important content.
- **End-of-Chapter Exercises and Practice Exercises:** Direct you to *use* content, helping you clarify understanding and move information into long-term memory.

Other Features You Need to Know About

- **Glossary:** Provides definitions of key terms. If you don't understand words, look them up, or you may miss major points.
- **Critical Moments:** Give simple strategies that can make a BIG difference in improving your efficiency and productivity.
- **Other Perspectives:** Offer interesting (and sometimes amusing) points of view encountered during manuscript preparation.

- **Response Key:** Example responses for End-of-Chapter Exercises and Practice Exercises are provided to help you evaluate your responses. This is called a *response key,* rather than an *answer key,* to avoid implying that there's *only one right answer* to each question. In many cases, a variety of responses are acceptable (great minds don't always think alike). The main point of the exercises isn't necessarily to come up with the right response: Rather, the point is to get in touch with the thinking that led you to your response, and to be able to evaluate and correct your thinking as needed.

Reading Efficiently

However you choose to read, keep in mind the following steps, which provide an organized and efficient way to master content.

- **Survey:** Scan the abstract, major headings, tables, and illustrations.
- **Question:** Turn major headings into questions.
- **Read:** Read, taking notes and answering your questions.
- **Review, Recite, and Re-read:** Review the chapter (or your notes), reciting key content out loud. Then ask yourself, "What's still not clear here?" Read the sections you don't understand again; raise questions to ask in class or discuss with your peers.

Acknowledgments

I want to thank my husband, Jim, for his love and support, and for being willing to hear the word *critical thinking* more than anyone in his right mind should ever have to. I also want to thank the rest of my family, and the following people for their belief in me, and their contribution to my personal and professional growth:

Emily Barrosse, Marty Kenney, Heidi Laird, Ledjie Ballard, Terri Patterson, Nancy Flynn, Carol Taylor, Connie Sechrist, Becky Resh, Diane Verity, Annette Sophocles, Barbara Cohen, Lynda and Richard Carpenito, Nat and Louise Rochester, Charlie and Nancy Lindsay, Mary Jo Boyer, John Payne, the Villanova College of Nursing Faculty, and the past and present staff nurses of Paoli Memorial Hospital.

I'm most grateful for the generous assistance of Leslie D. Gundry, Librarian, Pew Library of Bryn Mawr Hospital.

My *special thanks* go to the following people at W.B. Saunders: Thomas Eoyang, Vice President and Editor-in-Chief, Nursing Books, for his belief in this project, consistent support, and high standards; Barbara Cullen, Acquisitions Editor, who was sure there was a book just waiting to happen; I. Stacey Polk, Editorial Assistant, and Cass Stamato, Staff Support Specialist, for their support, sense of humor, and attention to detail; John Cooke, Executive Vice President, Production Services, for creating a vision of what can happen in production; Joan Wendt, Book Designer, whose "manuscript makeover magic" dressed this book for success; Tom Stringer, Copy Editing Supervisor, who readily grasped my intent and made copy editing checks a breeze; Linda R. Garber, Production Manager, for keeping us all on track; and Maura Connor, Marketing Manager, and the sales and marketing staff for their crucial role in making this book successful.

ROSALINDA ALFARO-LEFEVRE

Contents

CHAPTER 5
PRACTICAL CRITICAL THINKING SKILLS............92

RESPONSE KEY............136

Introduction

Assumptions and Promises

Before I began to write this book, I made some assumptions:

- You want to learn.
- Your time is valuable, and you don't want to waste it.
- You like to learn the most important things first.
- You learn better when you're motivated, know why information is relevant, and choose your own way of learning.
- It's inappropriate for *me* to tell *you* how to think.

- You feel a sense of accomplishment when you've mastered information that helps you be more independent.

Because of these assumptions, I promise to:

- Let you know what's most important.
- Provide the "reasons behind the rules."
- Encourage you to *choose* what works for *you*.
- Use lots of examples to make the information real.
- Help you gain or refine the skills required to be a better thinker, independent learner, and more effective nurse.

Four Ways We Change

This book is designed to help you develop and refine your thinking skills. This implies that I expect you'll make some changes. However, I must point out that modifying your thinking doesn't necessarily mean making *radical* changes. It usually means *becoming aware of how you think,* and making *small* changes that can really improve your efficiency and effectiveness. Take a moment to review the box Four Ways We Change, which addresses four ways we change and offers a way of changing that makes transitions easier. It's my hope that once you've reviewed this information, you'll be able to make changes with more confidence and less stress.

▶ Four Ways We Change*

1. Pendulum change:	"I was wrong before, but now I'm right."
2. Change by exception:	"I'm right, except for . . . ."
3. Incremental change:	"I was *almost* right before, but *now* I'm right."
4. Paradigm† change:	"What I knew before was *partially* right. What I know now is more right, but only part of what I'll know tomorrow."

▶ Paradigm Change Is Transformational

Paradigm change combines what's useful about *old ways* with what's useful about *new ways*, and keeps us open to looking for *even better* ways.

We realize:

- Our previous views were only part of the picture.
- What we now know is only part of what we'll know later.
- Change is no longer threatening: It enlarges and enriches.
- The unknown can then be friendly and interesting.
- Each insight smooths the road, making the change process easier.

---

*Adapted and summarized from Ferguson, M. (1980). *Aquarian conspiracy: Personal and social transformation in our time.* New York: G. P. Putnam's Sons.
†Pronounced pa'ra dīm.

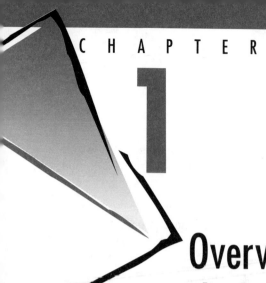

Overview: What Is Critical Thinking, and Why Is It Important?

T h i s   c h a p t e r   a t   a   g l a n c e .   .   .

PRE-CHAPTER SELF-TEST

Read the objectives listed below and decide whether you can readily achieve each one. If you can, you don't need to read this chapter and can go on to Chapter 2. Don't be concerned if you can't meet any of the objectives at this time. We'll come back to this self-test at the end of the chapter, so you'll get a second chance.

Suggestion: Mark your book or take notes when you encounter information that will help you achieve the objectives. Reading with a purpose is a key strategy that triggers your brain to get involved in what you're reading, carefully evaluating the material, and making decisions about what's important and how the material might be used.

O B J E C T I V E S

1. Define critical thinking using your own words, based on a commonly used definition of critical thinking.

2. Explain the difference between thinking and critical thinking.

3. Give three reasons why critical thinking is essential for nursing students.

4. Explain why it's important to be aware of how you think.

5. Describe five critical thinking characteristics you'd like to develop or improve.

6. Discuss how critical thinking is similar to, and different from, problem-solving.

7. Identify four principles of the scientific method that are evident in critical thinking.

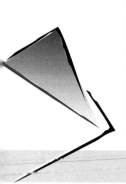

ABSTRACT

This chapter focuses on the big picture of critical thinking. It begins by considering critical thinking to be *highly developed thinking*, and addressing why teaching and learning critical thinking are essential. It then examines how this book helps develop thinking skills, and reinforces the need to gain awareness of how we think before trying to improve. Finally, it takes a closer look at critical thinking, asking you to consider questions like, "What's the difference between thinking and critical thinking?" "How is critical thinking commonly defined?" "What are characteristics of critical thinkers?" and "What's familiar and what's new about critical thinking?"

Why Focus on Critical Thinking?

The future belongs to those of us who learn to make the most of our brain power—those who *think critically*. To succeed in today's rapidly changing world, we must have more than current, job-specific knowledge. We need highly developed *thinking skills—critical thinking skills*—that help us adapt to new situations, make competent decisions, and teach ourselves.

We have at least four major motivating factors for teaching and learning critical thinking:

1. Critical thinking is the key to resolving problems. Nurses who don't think critically become part of the problems.
2. Nurses must make complex decisions, adapt to new situations, and continuously update their knowledge and skills. Critical thinking is integral to all of these.
3. Critical thinking will be essential to pass the National Council Licensure Examination (NCLEX).
4. National League for Nursing (NLN)–accredited programs must include content designed to develop critical thinking skills (see Display 1–1 NLN Statements on Critical Thinking).

How This Book Helps Develop Thinking Skills

Keeping the focus on concepts relevant to nursing, this book is designed to serve two major purposes:

1. To help you develop or refine habits that can make critical thinking more automatic.

Display 1-1	National League for Nursing (NLN) Statements on Critical Thinking

- Baccalaureate programs: "This outcome [critical thinking] reflects students' skills in reasoning, analysis, research or decision making relevant to the discipline of nursing" (NLN, 1991, p. 26).
- Associate degree programs: "The practice of a graduate from an associate degree nursing program is characterized by critical thinking" (NLN, 1990, p. 3).
- Diploma programs: "The graduate utilizes critical thinking in professional practice" (NLN, 1989, p. 2).

2. To encourage you to interact with the reading in a way that you'll be stimulated to *really think* about the content and how it applies to you. Critical thinking is active. You can't do it passively reading or listening to someone else's words. It has to happen in *your* brain. It requires interpreting information and answering questions like, "What does this really mean?" "How is this useful?" and "What are the implications of this?"

What's Your Thinking Style, and Why Does It Matter?

Having addressed the importance of getting involved in the reading, and deciding how information applies to you, I must reinforce a point made in the introduction: Improving thinking requires developing insight into how you think. Once you're aware of your thinking style—your usual approaches to gaining understanding and making decisions—and get in touch with your talents and blind spots, you can then find ways to improve.

Putting how we think *into words* isn't easy. In the past, we've rarely been asked to explain what goes on inside our heads as we think, and few of us have had the opportunity to *hear how others think*. However, this is changing. Experts are finding ways to help us put *how we think* into words. Once we can talk about how we think, we can then exchange information with others, learn strategies that make thinking more efficient, and practice to improve.

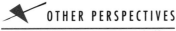 OTHER PERSPECTIVES

On Creativity and Appreciation of Effort
I'd rather have a basket of dandelions fresh-picked by a child, than the most beautiful bouquet of roses.
    Susan Giedgowd

There are numerous tests available for gaining insight and learning to talk about our thinking styles. Because we're still in the early stages of developing these tests, there's little known about their validity. For example, if you test out to be an *intuitive* person, we still don't know if you really *are* intuitive. However, most experts agree that even if we don't know much about the tests' validity, they're valuable tools for learning about ourselves and others.

While we won't take the time to actually take a thinking style test, take a few minutes to study Table 1–1, which gives some examples of various thinking styles. Which style (or styles) best describes *you*? Do you connect with any of them? Do you connect with more than one? Mark the one(s) that seems to best describe you, or add your own description—and remember there's *no right answer*. One style *isn't* better than another. They're all equally effective. The *best style* is the one that works for *you*.

If you were unaware of your thinking style, studying Table 1–1 should have given you a *beginning awareness* of how you think, and how other people think. As you read the following chapters, I hope you'll continue to develop insight and find ways to improve. Thinking is like any other skill (music, art, athletics). We each have our own styles and innate or learned capabilities. And we can all get better by gaining awareness, acquiring instruction, and consciously practicing to improve. Just as a tennis player practices strokes that make his game better, you must decide what thinking strategies work best for you, and use them to improve.

Table 1–1

EXAMPLES OF THINKING STYLES

Extrovert	Introvert
Thinks out loud	Thinks inside
Draws energy from being with people	Draws energy from being quiet
Sensate	Intuitive
Perceives the world discretely through the five senses	Perceives the world overall
Looks for facts	Looks for meaning
Thinking	Feeling
Uses objective data	Uses subjective data
Seeks just decisions	Seeks fair decisions
Judging	Perceiving
Orders the environment	Keeps things flexible and open
Likes to plan	Likes to be spontaneous

From Myers-Briggs Type Indicator (Myers, 1987). From Schoessler, M., Conedera, F., Bell, L., et al. (1993). Use of the Myers-Briggs type indicator to develop a continuing education department. *Journal of Nursing Staff Development*, 9 (1), 9.

OTHER PERSPECTIVES

Critical Thinking Can Be Triggered by Events that Are Fulfilling, as Well as Events that Are Problematic

When a baby is born at Bristol Hospital in Connecticut, everybody shares in the celebration. With each birth, the hospital's public address system plays the soothing strains of Brahm's Lullaby. Jean Young, the hospital's ICU patient care manager, says the tune brings smiles to the faces of everyone as they pause and reflect on the joy a new life brings.

"Patients especially love it," says Young, who learned about the program at the American Association of Critical-Care Nurses' National Teaching Institute and Critical Care Exposition. "Our outpatient oncology patients have had the most glowing remarks about the music's positive impact on them," she explains. "It lifts their spirits and takes their attention off themselves. It allows them to share someone else's joy and gives them something other than their hardships to think about."

Young notes that, at first, staff were uncertain about implementing the program. "There was always this concern about how it would be received by the poor mother and father who had just lost their baby. We decided we would give these parents the option of playing the lullaby or not. And, to this day, we have not encountered any adverse reception from the families. People who have had the program in place at other hospitals have said the same thing—that many of these parents want the lullaby played for their baby."

Young hopes other hospitals consider implementing this program. "It's such a simple thing we can do for patients and families that costs virtually nothing and brings a great deal of pleasure."

Reprinted from the August 1994 issue of AACN News with permission of the American Association of Critical-Care Nurses, Aliso Viejo, California.

What's the Difference Between Thinking and Critical Thinking?

Consider the following scenarios:

Scenario One ■ It's Tuesday. You're driving down the highway and the following is going through your mind: "I'll sure be glad when this week is over. I have so much to do . . . anatomy test on Wednesday . . . paper due on Thursday . . . work, tonight. . . . I really wanted to get a hair cut. . . . Do I really have to shop tomorrow? . . . Gee, what an interesting looking man that is on the corner. . . . I'm starving . . . what can I eat?"

Scenario Two ■ It's Wednesday, and you're taking the anatomy test. You're completely surprised by one of the questions. Your stomach turns into a knot, and you think, "I don't have a clue what this answer is. . . . I can't believe I don't know this. . . . I studied hard, but I don't remember this. . . . I can't believe it. . . . When did we talk about this? . . . We never covered this, did we? . . . I've got to get myself together and think . . . hmmm . . . think, think, think. If I could only think . . . Ten more minutes . . . I've got to get thinking . . . . I hate when this happens."

Scenario Three ■ It's Friday. You've had a bad week. The anatomy test was terrible. You were stressed out at work because you were worried about your paper. You finished your paper in a last-minute rush. You look ahead and feel overwhelmed with assignments and commitments. You think to yourself, "I've got to get organized. Tomorrow morning, I'm going to sit down with my calendar and figure out what I've got to do and when I'm going to do it. I'm going to write everything down, set priorities, and make up a schedule so I have some control over my life."

In all of the previous scenarios, you're thinking, right? Well, if you consider thinking to be any mental activity, you are. But look at Scenarios One and Two again. **Scenario One** shows aimless, passive thinking with ideas and images drifting through your head. **Scenario Two** shows attempts to begin active thinking to answer the question on the anatomy test, but your mind is stuck on negative thoughts that are getting you nowhere. **Scenario Three** shows focused, deliberate thought. You recognize your brain is overwhelmed with too much going on, and you take control, get organized, and take steps to make the most of your brain power. You're beginning to think critically.

So, what's the difference between thinking and critical thinking? The key difference is control. Thinking is basically any mental activity—it can be aimless and uncontrolled. It may serve a purpose, but we often aren't aware of its benefits. We might not even remember our thoughts at all. On the other hand, critical thinking is controlled, purposeful, and more likely to lead to obvious beneficial results.

Critical Thinking: Some Different Definitions

So then, how is *critical thinking* defined? First, I'll give you a one-word answer; then we'll look at some commonly used definitions.

A Synonym

If you ever hear, "Give me one word that explains critical thinking," the best word to offer is *reasoning*. If you were in elementary school today, you'd be learning "4 R's" instead of three: Reading, 'Riting, 'Rithmetic, and R*easoning*. Beginning in kindergarten, children are learning the *how to's* of effective reasoning (e.g., how to gain insight to solve problems and make wise decisions). This "fourth R" continues to be stressed throughout the primary and secondary schools. Tomorrow's world will be full of people who learned *reasoning skills,* or critical thinking skills, from a very early age.

Reasoning—now you have a synonym for critical thinking. However, because reasoning is a highly individualized, complex activity that involves *distinct ideas, emotions, and perceptions*, let's move on to a more substantial discussion.

Common Definitions

There are numerous definitions of critical thinking, from "reasonable reflective thinking that's focused on what to believe or do" (Ennis, 1987) to "the propensity to engage in an activity with reflective skepticism" (McPeck, 1981). Halpern (1984) described critical thinking as "purposeful, goal-directed thinking." For those of you who want more, additional definitions are listed in Appendix A.

An Applied Definition for Nursing

In search of a definition that's useful in describing nursing's critical thinking, I reviewed the literature, considered today's nursing roles, and developed the following definition, based on Halpern's work:

Unlike the "mindless" thinking we do when going about our daily routines, *critical thinking is purposeful, goal-directed thinking* that aims to make judgments based on evidence (fact), rather than conjecture (guesswork). *Based on principles of science and the scientific method* (e.g., maintaining a questioning attitude, following an organized approach to discovery, and making sure information is reliable), critical thinking requires developing strategies that *maximize* human potential (e.g., tapping on individual strengths) and *compensate* for problems caused by *human nature* (e.g., the powerful influence of personal perceptions, values, and beliefs).

To summarize, *critical thinking* in nursing:

- Entails purposeful, goal-directed thinking
- Aims to make judgments based on evidence (fact) rather than conjecture (guesswork)
- Is based on principles of science and scientific method
- Requires strategies that maximize *human potential* and compensate for problems caused by *human nature*

Characteristics (Attitudes) of Critical Thinkers

Some experts say that it's better to *describe* critical thinking than to *define* it: If you consider the characteristics, or attitudes, of those who consistently demonstrate critical thinking, you have an overall picture of what it takes to think critically. Consider Display 1–2, which provides a list of characteristics of critical thinkers: Compare yourself with each quality described, put a "W" next to the ones you feel you've developed *well,* and put an "I" next to those you'd like to *improve.* Then read on for a critique of this exercise.

If you had the *perfect role model critical thinker,* you'd have someone who demonstrated all of the qualities listed in Display 1–2. However, we all know that there's no such thing as a *perfect role model.* In fact, some of the best minds are tempted to mark that they'd like to improve almost all their characteristics (critical thinkers believe there's always room for improvement). If you weren't *tempted* to put at least a few "I's" above, it's likely that you need to give this activity more thought. Go back and do it again, identifying at least five qualities you'd like to improve.

| **Display 1–2** | **Characteristics (Attitudes) of Critical Thinkers** |

Critical thinkers are:

- **Active thinkers,** maintaining a questioning attitude, and double-checking both the reliability of information and their interpretation of the information.
- **Knowledgeable of their biases and limitations.** Some call this "having intellectual humility."*
- **Fair-minded,** keenly aware of the powerful influence of their own perceptions, values, and beliefs, but seeking to treat all viewpoints alike.
- **Willing to exert a conscious effort to work in a planful manner,** gathering information, checking for accuracy, and *persisting*, even when solutions aren't obvious or require several steps.
- **Good communicators,** realizing that *mutual exchange of ideas* is essential to understanding the facts and finding the best solutions.
- **Empathetic,** putting their own feelings aside, and consciously imagining themselves in the place of others in order to genuinely understand them. Some call this "having intellectual empathy."*
- **Open-minded,** willing to consider other perspectives and suspending judgment until all the evidence is weighed.
- **Independent thinkers,** making their own judgments and decisions, rather than allowing others to do it for them.
- **Curious and insightful,** questioning deeply, and interested in understanding underlying thoughts and feelings.
- **Humble,** recognizing that no one, including themselves, has all the answers or is immune to error.
- **Honest with themselves and others, admitting when their thinking may be flawed or requires more thought.** Some call this "having intellectual integrity."*
- **Proactive,** instead of *reactive*, anticipating problems and acting *before* they occur.
- **Organized and systematic in their approach** to solving problems and making decisions.
- **Flexible,** able to explore and imagine alternatives, and change approaches and priorities as needed.
- **Cognizant of rules of logic,** recognizing the role of intuition, but seeking evidence and weighing risks and benefits before acting.
- **Realistic,** acknowledging that we don't live in a perfect world, and that the best answers aren't always the perfect answers.
- **Team players,** willing to collaborate to work toward common goals.
- **Creative and committed to excellence,** continually evaluating; seeking clarity and accuracy, and looking for ways to improve how things get done.

---

*These terms originally came from Richard Paul (1993).

Reflection and Insight ("Hemming and Hawing" and "AHA!")

Once I asked a student how she went about answering test questions. She replied, "Usually I read the question, then I 'hem and haw' about what's being asked and what's the best response." Critical thinking requires reasonable, reflective thinking—it may require you to "hem and haw."

Another expression that describes critical thinking is "AHA!" We say "AHA!" when we suddenly realize something, or have our suspicions confirmed. We say "AHA!" when we connect with something that was in the back of our minds, but we had never put it into words—when our gut feelings tell us something is right. The "AHA!" experience is suddenly gaining awareness or insight into something we're trying to understand.

I hope as you read this book, you do a lot of "hemming and hawing" (reflecting) about what you read. If you're not sure about something or want to give it more thought, write a brief question in the margin or on a piece of paper, to remind yourself to come back to it. Then discuss your thoughts with a teacher or someone else. You'll be surprised how much more you'll gain from your reading—discussing key questions with others helps you clarify your thoughts, broaden your perspectives, and *understand and retain* what you read. I also hope you find "AHA's" as you read. These moments of "light bulbs going off in your head" are energizing. They often bring you new ideas, build your confidence, and stimulate you to learn more.

What's Familiar and What's New About Critical Thinking?

We understand something new best by comparing it with something we already know: How is it the same, and how is it different? This section first addresses critical thinking concepts you're likely to find familiar; then it addresses concepts that are likely to be new.

What's Familiar

Problem-solving. If you have sound problem-solving skills, you already know a lot about critical thinking. In many ways, critical thinking is like an "upgraded version" of the problem-solving method. Let me explain further. In the past, the problem-solving method has been viewed as the key to finding effective solutions. More recently, we've begun to realize the limitations of the problem-solving method. For example, it *starts* with a problem and *ends* with a solution. Critical thinking, on the other hand, is more *open-ended,* focusing on *continuous improvement,* regardless of whether or not problems exist.

I can almost hear some of you thinking, "But problem-solving is open-ended too, if you do it right. This 'critical thinking stuff' sounds just like good problem-solving to me." In many ways, critical thinking *is* simply good problem-solving.

However, there's at least one thing about critical thinking that's significantly different from problem-solving: Critical thinking may be triggered by positive events. For example, we see something good happen, and we think, "Hey! That's great!" If we're critical thinkers, we should be thinking, "We need to see if we can make this happen more frequently (or for everybody)." If we stayed in our "problem-solving mode," we might miss these positive triggers, and lose opportunities to progress.

To summarize: There's a trend to replace the term *problem solving* (because it implies all you're doing is solving problems) with *critical thinking* (because it implies you're doing more than problem-solving). This doesn't mean the term *problem-solving* is obsolete. It's still used and useful. However, if you're doing more than solving problems (if you're also preventing problems and maximizing potential and efficiency), use the term *critical thinking*.

The Scientific Method. There's a lot about critical thinking that you'll find similar to principles of science and the scientific method. For simplicity's sake, these are summarized in Display 1–3.

By now you might be thinking, "I already know most of this stuff." If so, that's great, because there's lot's new ahead as researchers increase our knowledge on maximizing human potential. Read on, and you'll see what I mean.

Display 1–3	Principles of Critical Thinking Similar to Principles of Science and the Scientific Method*

1. **Observing.** Continuously practicing observation and examination to gain understanding.
2. **Classifying data.** Grouping related information in order to reveal relationships among the observed facts.
3. **Drawing conclusions that follow logically.** ("If this is so, then . . . ")
4. **Conducting experiments.** Performing studies to gain understanding and identify ways of progressing.
5. **Testing hypotheses.** Determining whether the evidence supports what we *believe* to be true *is* true.

---

*It's important to recognize that some of us learned the scientific method as being a rigorous procedure that includes the study of hypotheses, theories, laws, and methods of exploration. Most now regard the scientific method as being *a family of methods for exploration*, with methods *differing* according to subject matter.

What's New

Maximizing Human Potential. This is the *Decade of the Brain*. We're only just beginning to learn how to tap the human potential to think critically. As we learn more, we can expect old theories and accepted ways of thinking to be challenged, modified, and sometimes replaced by newer, more effective ways of using our brains. For example, as

Display 1–4	What's New About Critical Thinking

- Research findings suggesting that intelligence quotient (IQ) tests may not really measure IQ, and that there are other focuses of intelligence (e.g., interpersonal intelligence) that influence our ability to think critically (Gardner, 1993; Jenks, 1993).
- The idea that thinking can and must be taught; that practicing thinking skills helps us be better thinkers.
- Information from the disciplines of neurology and neurosurgery suggesting that the brain is like a muscle: The more you use it, the more capable it becomes.
- The identification of new ways of stimulating interaction with information (during reading, lectures, and group discussions) to enhance learning and understanding: Critical thinking is *active*, rather than passive.
- The belief that personal interests, passions, and commitments, as well as a sense of esthetics (beauty), mystery, and wonder, play a crucial role in developing *attitudes* necessary for thinking.
- Increased concern about the *process* of reasoning: It's often as important to know *how* a conclusion or decision is made, as it is to know *what* the conclusion or decision is.
- Greater emphasis on *understanding other perspectives*, *using* several *different perspectives* (collaborating) to enhance ability to reason. In other words, great minds don't always think alike: Different viewpoints enhance our thinking.
- More acceptance of "There's more than one way" and sometimes there are "no *right* answers" (each answer is correct in its own way).
- Increased acknowledgment that there are *useful mistakes* (occasional failure is the price of improvement), and that *sharing mistakes* is a responsible action that helps others avoid the same errors.
- More research on finding ways of "measuring" how someone thinks (new and better testing methods).
- The identification of strategies that help us compensate for problems created by *human nature* (we tend to see what we *expect* to see, what's familiar; we're influenced by personal values and beliefs; we resist change; we like being right).
- The identification of strategies that help us take advantage of how our brains work, including how to:
  - Get information into long-term memory
  - Form good habits of inquiry
  - Enhance creativity

youngsters, we were all encouraged to memorize. However, few of us learned *how to memorize* in a way that promotes comprehension and retention. We simply tried to memorize facts. We now know that memorizing a list of facts can be a dead end for our minds—it doesn't help us *understand* information, and it doesn't help us *remember it in the long term*. We're beginning to identify strategies like using visual centers of the brain, and using preferred learning styles to promote understanding and retention. We'll examine how to use these and other strategies in later chapters, but for now, look at Display 1–4, which gives an overview of what's new in critical thinking.

Summary

By now, you should have an idea of *what* critical thinking is, and *why* it's important. To solidify your understanding, review the following *Key Points,* and then complete the end-of-chapter exercises. Once you've done that, you'll be ready to go on to the next chapter, which addresses *how* to improve your thinking.

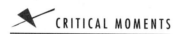

CRITICAL MOMENTS

Critical thinkers are self-assessing, self-examining, and self-improving. Take a few moments every week to evaluate how your life is going and identify ways to improve. Have you ever known anyone who improved at anything without working at it?

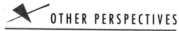

CRITICAL MOMENTS

Socrates learned more from questioning others than he did from reading books. Seek others' opinions, and question deeply to gain understanding.

OTHER PERSPECTIVES

Always Thinking!

One night I was helping my third-grade son with his English assignment.
"What is a noun?" I asked.
"A person, place, or thing," he replied.
I then asked, "What is a pronoun?"
I could see the wheels turning in his head before he answered, "A really good noun."

Contributed by Mike Collins. Reprinted with permission from the June 1993 Readers Digest. Copyright © 1993 by the Readers Digest Assn., Inc.

KEY POINTS

▶ To succeed in today's rapidly changing world, we need highly developed thinking skills—*critical thinking skills*—that help us adapt to new situations, make competent decisions, and teach ourselves.

▶ Critical thinking is the key to resolving problems. Nurses who don't think critically become *part* of the problems.

▶ Thinking is like any other skill (music, art, athletics). We each have our own styles and innate or learned capabilities. And we can all improve by gaining awareness acquiring instruction, and consciously practicing to improve.

▶ *Thinking* is basically any *mental activity*—it can be aimless and uncontrolled. *Critical thinking* is controlled, purposeful, and more likely to lead to obvious beneficial results.

▶ *Reasoning* is a good synonym for critical thinking: If you were in elementary school today, you'd be learning "4 R's": Reading, 'Riting, 'Rithmetic, and Reasoning.

▶ Reasoning is a highly individualized, complex activity that involves distinct ideas, emotions, and perceptions.

▶ Page 9 provides some common definitions of critical thinking and an applied definition for nursing.

▶ If you consider the characteristics, or attitudes, of those who consistently demonstrate critical thinking, you have an overall picture of what it takes to think critically (see Display 1–2 on page 10).

▶ Critical thinking requires reasonable, reflective thinking—it may require you to "hem and haw." The "AHA!" experience is suddenly gaining awareness or insight into something we're trying to understand.

▶ In many ways, critical thinking is like an "upgraded version" of the problem-solving method.

▶ Unlike the problem-solving method, critical thinking may be triggered by positive events: If we see something that works well, we need to start thinking about how to use it to our advantage.

▶ There's a trend to replace the term *problem-solving* (because it implies all you're doing is solving problems) with *critical thinking* (because it implies you're doing more than problem-solving).

▶ There's a lot about critical thinking that you'll find similar to principles of science and the scientific method (see Display 1–3 on page 12).

▶ This is the *Decade of the Brain*—we're only just beginning to learn how to tap the human potential to think critically. Display 1–4 on page 13 gives an overview of what's new about critical thinking.

▶ Figure 1–1 on page 16 provides a "visual summary" of questions you should consider to evaluate your potential to think critically.

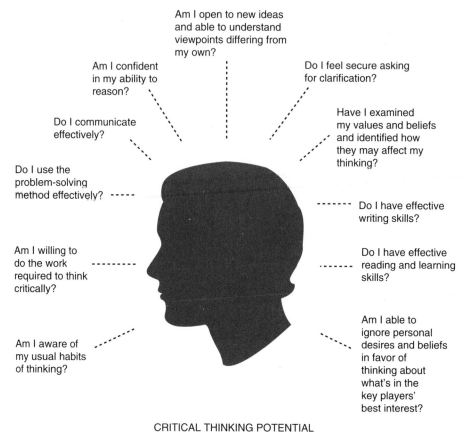

Am I open to new ideas and able to understand viewpoints differing from my own?

Am I confident in my ability to reason?

Do I feel secure asking for clarification?

Do I communicate effectively?

Have I examined my values and beliefs and identified how they may affect my thinking?

Do I use the problem-solving method effectively?

Do I have effective writing skills?

Am I willing to do the work required to think critically?

Do I have effective reading and learning skills?

Am I aware of my usual habits of thinking?

Am I able to ignore personal desires and beliefs in favor of thinking about what's in the key players' best interest?

CRITICAL THINKING POTENTIAL

Figure 1–1
Questions to ask yourself to evaluate your potential to think critically.

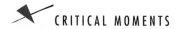 **CRITICAL MOMENTS**

A wise man changes his mind; a fool never will.
> Spanish proverb.

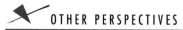 **OTHER PERSPECTIVES**

In Teamwork and Collaboration, Everyone Counts!

My night flight from Washington, D.C., was uneventful until we landed in Indianapolis. The plane was taxiing to the terminal but stopped in the middle of the runway. Many passengers were beginning to fidget in their seats as the engines idled. Then the pilot made an announcement that defused the tension: "I flew this multimillion-dollar aircraft from Washington, D.C., at night and found the airport on my first try. However, I have to wait until a guy with a couple of 99-cent flashlights shows me how to park it."

Contributed by Richard L. Smuck. Reprinted with permission from the July 1994 Readers Digest. Copyright © 1994 by the Readers Digest Assn., Inc.

■■■ RECOMMENDATIONS FOR COMPLETING THE END-OF-CHAPTER EXERCISES

1. Keep a record of your responses. Choose a notebook you *like* using, or use a computer. I like using a loose-leaf notebook because you can easily remove, add, or replace pages. Keeping all your responses together will give you a record you can review later to see how you've progressed. Since we'll go from simple to more complex ideas, you'll be surprised at the progress that will be evident when you review your responses later on.
2. At first, be more concerned with *substance* than grammar (like you would if you were writing a diary). However, as you progress, work to make your responses *clear to others*. Making your responses clear to others will help you clarify your thoughts.
3. Keep it legible: Print, if you must. Use a number two pencil if you tend to make a lot of changes.
4. If you have trouble *writing*, and do better *verbally,* tape your response, then record it. This will save you time in the long run.
5. Don't be afraid to paraphrase: Paraphrasing helps you gain understanding because you explain what you read using familiar language (your own). To avoid concerns of plagiarism, cite the page numbers that you've chosen to paraphrase.

End-of-Chapter Exercises

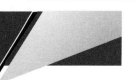

Instructions:

Limit responses to 2–5 sentences.

1. The introduction on page 1 discusses four ways we change, and offers a way of making changes less stressful. Complete the following:
   a. When I make changes, I usually . . . .
   b. I would like to improve my ability to adapt to change by . . . .
2. Complete the following: If I were to tell someone how I think, I would say that I . . . .
3. Complete the pre-chapter self-test, which has been reproduced below:
   a. Define critical thinking using your own words, based on a commonly used definition of critical thinking.*
   b. Explain the difference between thinking and critical thinking.*
   c. Give three reasons why critical thinking is essential for nursing students.*
   d. Explain why it's important to be aware of how you think.*
   e. Describe five critical thinking characteristics you'd like to develop or improve.*
   f. Discuss how critical thinking is similar to, and different from, problem-solving.*
   g. Identify four principles of the scientific method that are evident in critical thinking.*

---

*An *example response* for this exercise can be found in the *Response Key* at the back of the book beginning on page 136.

2

How to Think Critically

Why Read This Chapter?

PRE-CHAPTER SELF-TEST

Read the objectives listed below and decide whether you can readily achieve each one. If you can, skip this chapter, and go on to Chapter 3. Don't be concerned if you can't meet any of the objectives at this time. We'll come back to this self-test at the end of the chapter, so you'll get a second chance.

O B J E C T I V E S

1. Address five factors that influence critical thinking and explain how or why each one is influential.

2. Explain how human habits can influence critical thinking ability.

3. Give five practical strategies that can enhance critical thinking, and explain why the strategies work.

4. Explain why developing effective interpersonal and communication skills is essential to critical thinking.

5. Identify the roles of logic, intuition, and trial-and-error in critical thinking.

6. Discuss at least five critical thinking skills you'd like to improve, and how you intend to improve them.

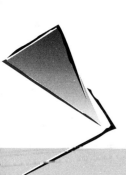

A B S T R A C T

This chapter addresses how to develop strategies for critical thinking. It examines factors influencing critical thinking, stressing that being aware of how and why these factors are so influential helps us identify strategies to improve. Communication techniques that facilitate critical thinking are presented, and the roles of logic, intuition, and trial-and-error in critical thinking are discussed. Finally, it gives *specific* critical thinking strategies, and addresses *skills* that should be mastered to be able to think critically.

Chapter 1 focused on *what* critical thinking is and *why* it's important. This chapter focuses on *how* to think critically. We've already addressed the need to gain awareness of how we think so that we can identify ways of improving. Now let's look at some factors that *affect* how we think. Once we're aware of what these factors are, and how we're influenced by them, we can then develop strategies to increase our ability to think critically in various situations.

Factors Influencing Critical Thinking Ability

Have you ever found yourself saying, "I just wasn't thinking right"? Or, better, "Boy, that really got me thinking—I came up with some great ideas!" We've all felt this way at one time or another. Our ability to think well varies, depending on personal factors, and circumstances that are evident at the time. For example, look at Table 2–1, which lists factors usually enhancing critical thinking and those usually impeding critical thinking. Then read on for an explanation of *how and why* these factors are so influential.

Personal Factors

Moral Development (Fairmindedness). Many experts cite a positive correlation between moral development and critical thinking ability: People with a mature level of moral development—those with a clear, carefully reasoned sense of *what's right, wrong, and fair*—are more likely to think critically. It makes sense that those who are keenly aware of their values and beliefs, and who approach situations with an attitude of "I must consider all viewpoints and make decisions that are *in the key players' best interest,*" have already developed critical thinking habits.

Table 2-1

FACTORS INFLUENCING CRITICAL THINKING

Factors *Usually **Enhancing*** Critical Thinking	Factors *Usually **Impeding*** Critical Thinking
Personal Factors	**Personal Factors**
Moral development (fairmindedness)	Dislikes, prejudices, biases
Age (older you are)	Lack of self-confidence
Self-confidence*	Limited knowledge of problem-solving,
Knowledge of problem-solving, decision-making, and research principles	decision-making, and research principles
	Poor communication skills
Effective communication and interpersonal skills	Limited early evaluation
	Poor writing skills
Habitual early evaluation	Poor reading and learning skills
Past experience*	
Effective writing skills	**Situational Factors**
Effective reading and learning skills	Anxiety†/stress/fatigue
	Emotional extremes (anger, joy)
Situational Factors	Lack of motivation
Knowledge of related factors	Limited knowledge of related factors
Awareness of resources	Lack of awareness of resources
Awareness of risks*	Time limitations†
Positive reinforcement	Environmental distractions
Presence of motivating factors	

* Sometimes may *impede* critical thinking (see text on pages 20–24).
† Sometimes may *enhance* critical thinking (see text on pages 20–24).

Age. Most authors agree that age also correlates with critical thinking ability: Older people are more likely to be critical thinkers. There are two logical reasons for this: (1) Moral development usually comes with maturity. (2) Most older people have had more opportunities to practice reasoning in different situations.

Dislikes, Prejudices, and Biases. These are often subtle, but almost always powerful factors that *hinder* critical thinking. If you're unable to recognize and overcome these factors, it will be difficult to think critically in situations where you have to function in spite of your dislikes, prejudices, and biases.

Self-confidence. For the most part, self-confidence aids critical thinking. If we aren't confident, we use much of our brain power worrying about failure, reducing the energy available for *productive thinking*. Occasionally, self-confidence is an *impeding* factor: Some become so *overly confident* that they believe they can't be wrong, or that they have little to learn from others.

Knowledge of Problem-solving, Decision-making, Nursing Process, and Research Principles. Because critical thinking is based on many of the same principles, familiarity with the these methods *enhances* critical thinking.

Effective Communication and Interpersonal Skills. Developing effective communication and interpersonal skills is essential to critical thinking. We must be able to understand others, be understood by others, and gain others' trust to get the *facts* required for sound reasoning. Keep in mind that communication is more than talking and listening: We need to consider the messages we send by our *behavior* over a period of time. For example, to develop good interpersonal relationships, we need to demonstrate behaviors that send messages like, "I respect you," "I can be trusted," and "I want to do a good job."

Habitual Early Evaluation. When we evaluate early, checking whether our information is accurate, complete, and up-to-date, we're able to make corrections *early.* We avoid making decisions based on outdated, inaccurate, or incomplete information. Early evaluation enhances our ability to act safely and effectively. It improves our *efficiency* by helping us stay focused on priorities and avoid wasting time continuing useless actions. When we evaluate early by comparing our progress with a written plan, we are better able to stay on our intended path of thought—our brains often don't notice when we've "gone off on a tangent." For example, if I hadn't consistently checked to be sure that I followed the plan I developed for this book, I can assure you, you'd be reading some lengthy sections that would be interesting to *me,* but irrelevant and boring for *you!*

Past Experience. Most authors view this as an *enhancing* factor: Experienced nurses are usually better able to think critically because they have previous job-specific and problem-solving knowledge. However, sometimes, past experience is an *impeding* factor: We become victims of "tunnel vision," seeing only what we expect to see. If our past experience is *different* from the present situation, we may have trouble thinking critically. A classic example of this is when a nurse with *psychiatric expertise* fails to consider whether someone's confusion could be related to a *medical problem,* and vice versa (a nurse with *medical expertise* fails to consider whether someone's confusion could be related to a *psychiatric problem).*

Effective Writing Skills. These *promote* critical thinking. When we learn how to make ourselves clear in writing, we learn to apply critical thinking principles like identifying an organized approach, deciding what's relevant, focusing on others' perspectives, and clarifying our thoughts. Appendix C on page 150 provides strategies for improving writing skills.

Effective Reading and Learning Skills. These are *enhancing* factors. Critical thinking often requires us to use resources independently— we must know how to read and learn well. Having effective reading skills doesn't mean knowing how to read *rapidly.* It means taking the time to identify what's important, draw conclusions about what the material implies, and consider how it applies to the real world. Developing effective learning skills requires awareness of preferred learning styles, and using strategies that help us learn more easily by using *our preferred styles.* (See Appendix B on page 147 for examples of preferred learning styles and corresponding useful strategies.)

Situational Factors

Anxiety/Stress/Fatigue. For the most part, these *reduce* our thinking power. High levels of anxiety and stress, often the first to tap our brain energy, make concentration difficult. When we're fatigued, we're already operating on a "low battery." However, a *low* anxiety level, like being a little nervous about a test, can *promote* critical thinking by motivating us to be prepared.

Emotional Extremes (Anger, Joy). These *impede* critical thinking. Emotional extremes tend to make us focus only on the facts that are congruent with our intense feeling (only the good if we're happy, only the bad if we're mad). Have you ever been so happy or mad that you made a decision you regretted?

Awareness of Risks Involved. Usually this is an *enhancing* factor. When we know the risks, we think more carefully, making sure we've made a prudent decision before acting. Sometimes, especially for beginning students, awareness of the risks can increase anxiety to a level that *impedes* critical thinking. Almost everyone can imagine how hard it is to think critically when giving an injection for the first time!

Knowledge of Related Factors. The more we know about a situation, the better we'll be able to reason. For example, we might know about *diabetes,* but if we also know the *person* we're going to teach—know the person's lifestyle, desires, and motivations—we'll be more likely to design a plan of care that the person is willing to follow.

Awareness of Resources. Awareness of *resources* allows us to think critically, even with limited knowledge. For example, nurses frequently think critically about drug administration with limited drug-specific knowledge. They check with resources like pharmacists and drug manuals before giving unfamiliar drugs (e.g., they find out usual dose range, contraindications, and possible side effects).

Positive Reinforcement. This *promotes* critical thinking by helping us build self-confidence and focus on what we're doing *right.*

Presence of Motivating Factors. Factors that motivate us to *want* to think critically aid our thinking because they connect with our *own desires,* enticing us to get our brain "in gear." It's important to remember that what motivates *us* might not motivate *someone else.* An example of a *common* motivating factor for critical thinking is knowing *why* you're asked to do or study something (knowing why the action is important, or knowing how it's useful).

Time Limitations. This can be an *enhancing or impeding* factor. Time limitations, *when realistic,* are motivating factors: Deadlines stimulate us to get going and get things done. However, if there's *too little time,* we may make decisions quicker than we'd like, and come up with less than satisfactory answers. It's interesting to note that the courts recognize time limitations as a factor that influences our thinking. Courts give more leeway when examining decisions that were made in emergency situations, than those made with plenty of time for thinking. They give less leeway when considering decisions made hastily, if there actually was plenty of time.

Environmental Distractions. These impede critical thinking for obvious reasons—the more distractions there are, the more difficult it is to stay focused.

Okay. We've now covered factors influencing critical thinking ability. However, I've saved a major factor for a separate discussion: The *human factor.*

As *humans,* we have many wonderful qualities—qualities that separate us from other life on this planet. However, as humans, we also instinctually develop habits that serve to help us feel better about ourselves—habits that protect us for the moment, but *in the long run* hinder our potential to think critically. Let's take a look at some of the more common human habits that create barriers to critical thinking.

Habits Causing Barriers to Critical Thinking

The most common habits causing barriers to critical thinking are the *mine-is-better habit,* the *choosing-only-one* habit, and the *face-saving, resistance to change, conformity, stereotyping,* and *self-deception* habits.* The following is a discussion of each of these habits. Consider each one in relation to yourself and others you know. As you do this, keep in mind that we're all human, and that most of these habits are simply a result of human nature. Whether we realize it or not, we're all victims of these behaviors to some extent at one time or another.

The Mine-Is-Better Habit. We all tend to regard our ideas, values, religions, cultures, and points of view as being superior to others. To enhance our potential for critical thinking, we need to consciously work to control this habit as we're searching for truth.

---

*These habits (except for the choosing-only-one habit, which has been added by the author) are summarized from THE ART OF THINKING: A GUIDE TO CRITICAL AND CREATIVE THOUGHT, 3rd Edition by Vincent Ryan Ruggiero. Copyright © 1991 by HarperCollins Publishers, Inc. Reprinted by permission.

The Choosing-Only-One Habit. When faced with two choices, we tend to choose *only one* of the two. We forget to think about things like, "Are there other, better choices? Can we do both? Can we do neither?" Beginners are usually the most vulnerable to the choosing-only-one habit. They tend to blindly accept that if they've chosen one of two choices, then they've made a good decision. They also tend to make the common assumption of, "There must be one best way to do this" rather than, "There probably are several good ways of doing this, and each has its advantages and disadvantages." We can overcome this tendency by remembering to ask ourselves, "Must I choose only one?" or "Is this the only way?"

Face-saving. When we find that we've done or said something wrong, we have a strong instinct to protect our image—we try to save face. Critical thinking requires us to learn and grow. As we learn and grow, we'll make mistakes or realize our old ways of thinking or doing things can be improved. To be a critical thinker, we must learn to be comfortable saying things like, "I was wrong" or "I changed my mind."

Resistance to Change. While most of us realize change usually occurs for very good reasons, we tend to resist it. All too often, change is considered "guilty until proven innocent." We reject new ideas and ways without examining them fairly. Overcoming this barrier doesn't mean embracing every new idea uncritically. It means being willing to suspend judgment long enough to make an informed decision on whether the change is worthwhile.

Conformity. While some conformity, like following policies and procedures, is good, we sometimes engage in *harmful conformity*. Harmful conformity is when we conform to group thinking, rather than *think independently,* to avoid being viewed as "different." Once we conform, we might not realize that we say and do only those things we believe *others expect,* stifling our ability to be creative and improve.

Stereotyping. We stereotype when we make fixed and unbending overgeneralizations about others (e.g., "homeless people aren't very bright"). When our minds are fixed and unbending, we'll be unlikely to see what's really before us. By recognizing our tendency to stereotype, we can make a conscious effort to overcome this pattern, which distorts our view of reality.

Self-deception. This is a common habit that can be a real "turn off" to others: It's the purposeful forgetting of things about ourselves we don't particularly feel good about. An example of this is when people, usually in a face-saving effort, pretend to be knowledgeable about something, and then begin to believe they are knowledgeable. Admitting, "You know, I don't know much about that . . . I have to find out" is a much better strategy in the long run. Who wants to rely on people who are unwilling to admit their limitations?

To summarize, being aware of habits and factors influencing critical thinking helps us identify strategies that promote critical thinking. For example, if we know anxiety and stress impede critical thinking, we know we need to *reduce anxiety and stress* to enhance critical thinking. As humans, we might all be victims of deeply ingrained habits of mine-is-better, choosing-only-one, resistance to change, face-saving, conformity, stereotyping, and self-deception. It's simply human nature. However, as humans, we can overcome these barriers by becoming aware of our human ways, and working to replace old patterns with new ways of responding.

Covey's Seven Habits of Highly Effective People

Steven Covey, author of the highly successful book *The Seven Habits of Highly Effective People* (1989), also addresses the importance of replacing old patterns with new habits. He offers seven habits that can help us be more effective in creating positive personal and professional relationships. These habits, summarized in Display 2–1, enhance critical thinking because, as addressed earlier, critical thinking depends on our ability to develop the interpersonal relationships required to gain information and work as a team.

Display 2–1 | **Covey's "The Seven Habits of Highly Effective People®"**

1. **Be Proactive.™** Choose to be responsible for your own life, anticipate responses, and act before things happen.
2. **Begin With the End in Mind.™** Develop goals and make your expectations explicit.
3. **Put First Things First.™** Decide what's important, and stick to priorities moment by moment, day by day.
4. **Think Win-Win.™** Seek *mutual benefit* in all human interactions.
5. **Seek First to Understand, Then to be Understood.™** Communicate effectively.
6. **Synergize.™** Recognize that the whole is greater than the sum of its parts: Collaborate, bringing diverse ideas and talents together to create new and better ideas.
7. **Sharpen the Saw.™** Look after yourself physically, emotionally, and spiritually. (Covey explains *Sharpening the Saw™* by telling a story about a man who is sawing a tree trunk for hours: The saw is dull, and the man is exhausted. Someone suggests that he might do better if he sharpens the saw. The man responds, "I don't have time," and continues to work ineffectively.)

Summarized from: Covey, S. © (1989). "*The Seven Habits of Highly Effective People.*" New York: Simon & Schuster. Used with permission of Covey Leadership, Inc. All trademarks of the Covey Leadership Inc. are used with permission. All rights reserved. 1-800-331-7716.

Communicating Effectively

As well as developing habits that promote positive interpersonal relationships, it's essential to develop strategies that help us communicate effectively: Critical thinking depends on *mutual exchange* of ideas. Take a few moments to study Display 2–2, which provides specific communication techniques that can enhance critical thinking.

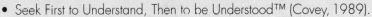

| Display 2–2 | Communication Strategies Enhancing Critical Thinking |

- Seek First to Understand, Then to be Understood™ (Covey, 1989).
- Clearly state that your intent is not to *judge*, but to *understand* (e.g., "I'm not here to judge. I just want to understand what's going on").
- Use strategies that help you see other points of view.
    - Ask for clarification. For example, "I don't mean to be difficult, but I still don't understand... can you clarify further?
    - Use phrases like "from your way of looking at it..." or "from your perspective...." For example, *"From your perspective,* how do you see this situation?"
    - Paraphrase in your own words. For example, "It seems to me that you're saying... Is that correct?"
    - Listen empathetically (with the intent of entering into the other person's way of looking at the world). This is often called trying to imagine what it would be like to "walk in another's shoes." Listening empathetically requires four steps: (1) Clear your mind of thoughts about how you view the situation or concerns about how you're going to respond. (2) Focus on listening to the person's feelings and perceptions. (3) Rephrase the feelings and perceptions as you understand them to be. (4) Detach, and come back to your own frame of reference.
- Apply strategies that help you get accurate and comprehensive information.
    - Use open-ended questions (those requiring more than a one-word answer). For example, "How do you feel about leaving tomorrow?"
    - Avoid closed-ended question (those requiring only a one-word answer). For example, "Are you ready to leave tomorrow?"
    - Use exploratory statements that lead the person to expand on certain issues. For example, "Tell me more about...."
    - Don't use leading questions (those that lead someone to a desired answer). For example, "You don't smoke, do you?"
    - Put body language into words. For example, "You looked a little sad...."
    - Use silence. Allow the person time to gather his thoughts.
- Remember the value of using written communication.
    - Record the information you gathered, then look to see what's missing and check for inconsistencies.
    - Ask the person to keep a log or diary, or keep one yourself.

Display continued on following page

Display 2-2	Communication Strategies Enhancing Critical Thinking (*Continued*)

- Apply strategies that help you get your point across.
  - Make sure the time and place are appropriate.
  - Wait until the person is ready to listen.
  - When voicing an opinion, use phrases that *convey* that you're *voicing an opinion*, rather than dictating what is so (e.g., "From my way of looking at it". . . ."From my perspective. . . .")
  - Ask the person to paraphrase what you've said (e.g., "I need to be sure you understand. Explain to me what I just said.").
- Demonstrate behaviors that help build positive interpersonal relationships.
  - Be cognizant of others' communication styles, rather than trying to force them to use yours (e.g., don't use touch, even if you like to. If the other person seems to recoil from touch; if someone is formal and reserved, respect his style).
  - Exhibit behaviors that send messages like, "I'm responsible," "I can be trusted," and "I want to do a good job." For example, keep promises, be punctual, accept responsibility, and respect others' time.
  - Acknowledge and apologize when you've caused inconvenience, been careless or made a mistake, or offended someone.
  - Respect others' territory, ask permission (e.g., "May I listen to your chest?" rather than, "Sit up, and let me listen to your chest").

Critical Thinking Strategies

Now that we've addressed factors influencing critical thinking (personal and situational factors, habits, and communication), let's go on to consider some *specific strategies* for promoting critical thinking.

Eight Key Questions

Have you ever heard the saying, "It's not what you know, but what you know to *ask*"? There are eight key questions that can help you determine your approach to critical thinking in different situations. These are summarized in Display 2–3 and addressed in more depth below.

1. **What's the goal of my thinking?** Clearly identifying our goal helps us be more focused and choose appropriate methods of achieving the goal. For example, consider how our approach differs if our goal is to get an "A" on a multiple choice test on IV therapy, compared with if the goal is to be prepared to care for someone with an IV line.
2. **What are the circumstances?** The approach to critical thinking varies, depending on the circumstances. For example, consider the following situation: You're in a classroom and the instructor asks you how you would manage a patient in shock. You aren't sure, but you *think* you know, so it's appropriate for you to answer. However, if

Display 2–3	**Eight Key Questions in Critical Thinking**

1. What's the goal of my thinking?
2. What are the circumstances?
3. What knowledge is required?
4. How much room is there for error?
5. How much time do I have?
6. What resources can help me?
7. Whose perspectives must be considered?
8. What's influencing my thinking?

you're in the clinical area, trying to manage this problem alone based on uncertain knowledge is inappropriate.

3. **What knowledge is required?** Discipline-specific knowledge is essential to being able to think critically. For example, how can we think critically about managing cardiac pain if we don't know the causes and common treatments of cardiac pain? If you don't know what knowledge is required, you probably don't know enough to achieve your goal—you need to get help.

4. **How much room is there for error?** When there's less room for error, we must carefully assess the situation, examine *all possible solutions,* and make every effort to make prudent decisions. For example, which situation below has less room for error, and how might your approach to decision-making differ in each situation?

   a. You're trying to decide whether to give an over-the-counter antihistamine to someone who's been in excellent health, but has been having trouble sleeping.

   b. You're trying to decide whether to give an over-the-counter antihistamine to someone with multiple health problems.

   Obviously, situation *a* has more room for error, because the person is healthy, therefore less likely to have pre-existing conditions that might be aggravated by the antihistamine. In situation *b,* unlike situation *a,* you need to consult the person's attending physician.

5. **How much time do I have?** If we have plenty of time to make a decision, we can take time to think independently, using resources such as textbooks to guide our thinking. If we don't have much time, we may be required to *refer* the problem to an expert immediately, to expedite care delivery.

6. **What resources can help me?** Identifying our resources (textbooks, computers, expert clinicians) is essential to accessing the information we need to be able to think critically. For example, most nurses don't know every hospital policy by heart. Rather, they know what situations are covered by policies, and refer to the policy manual as needed.

7. **Whose perspectives _must_ be considered?** Efficient solutions must consider the perspectives of all of the "key players" involved, or you risk having conflicting purposes. For example, to develop an effective plan for home care, the plan must consider the perspectives of patients, other household members, and other key members of the health care team. Imagine what could happen if you sent a grandmother home with lots of brightly colored medications, and everyone forgot to consider "the perspective" of a toddler in the home!

8. **What's influencing my thinking?** Recognizing influencing factors (e.g., personal beliefs and biases, previous bad experiences, fatigue) helps us gain objectivity and find ways to compensate for factors that might impede our ability to think clearly. For example, a nurse who is strongly against abortion would be wise to avoid working in gynecology, where women's decisions might make it difficult to give nursing care objectively.

Using Logic, Intuition, and Trial-and-Error

Depending on the situation, using logic, intuition, or trial-and-error is a common strategy for critical thinking. However, it's important to know when using each of these is _appropriate_. Using intuition or trial-and-error, _alone,_ is _risky:_ But if you use these two strategies together with logical thought, you can reduce the risks and use them effectively. Let's consider when and how to use logic, intuition, and trial-and-error.

- **Logic,** or sound reasoning that's based on evidence, is the foundation for critical thinking. It's the safest and most reliable strategy for problem-solving, and therefore should be used when making all important decisions.

- **Intuition** is best described as knowing something without evidence. The most effective use of intuition is to use it _as a guide to look for evidence._ For example, if your intuition tells you something is wrong with someone, you need to regard this feeling as a "red flag" that says "Watch this person closely" or "Get an expert here quickly to check this person." Using intuition is a valuable strategy for problem-solving, especially for experienced nurses, who may subconsciously recall a wide range of experiences. However, before you _act_ on intuition alone—before you act on gut feelings that aren't supported by evidence—be sure your actions won't cause harm.

- **Trial-and-error,** or trying several solutions until one that works is found, is a _risky_ but sometimes necessary approach to problem-solving. Trial-and-error should be used _only_ when there's plenty of room for error, when the problem can be monitored closely, and when the solutions have been logically thought through. An example of when trial-and-error is commonly used in nursing is in trying to determine the best way for a sterile dressing to be applied to an active person's wound: Often it takes several tries before the best way can be determined.

Focusing on the Big and Small Picture

There's a trend to emphasize the importance of focusing on the "big picture" (the whole) rather than the "small picture" (the parts). However, usually we need to do *both,* if we want to think critically. Consider the following scenarios.

Scenario One ■ Mr. Stevens is admitted to the hospital with a fractured pelvis. At the big-picture level, you need to develop long-term goals (e.g., *By day 7, Mr. Stevens will be discharged home ambulating independently with a walker*). At the small-picture level, you need to develop short-term goals (e.g., *By day 3, Mr. Stevens will be ambulating in physical therapy twice daily, using the walker with assistance*). Monitoring the small picture (whether Mr. Stevens is meeting short-term goals) helps you know if you're staying on schedule for the big picture (discharging Mr. Stevens by day 7).

Scenario Two ■ Mr. Juarez is in the coronary care unit, and tells you he's experiencing chest pain. Treating *both* "the whole" (Mr. Juarez's pain and anxiety) and "the parts" (Mr. Juarez's oxygen-deprived heart) is essential to resolving the chest pain (and, perhaps, to saving his life).

Scenario Three ■ You're trying to teach Tonya how to care for her newborn. You're well prepared with lots of nice pamphlets. She seems interested, but she keeps yawning and doesn't seem to retain information very long. Finally you say, "Is there a better time we could do this?" She admits that she hasn't slept all night and is extremely fatigued. You come back later after Tonya's had a good rest. She learns readily. In this case, paying attention to an important *detail* (the fact that she was tired) helped you be a more effective teacher.

To improve your ability to think critically, remember to ask questions like, "What's the big picture here?" "What's the small picture here?" "Am I considering both the parts and the whole?" and "Am I paying attention to key details?"

Specific Strategies

Several authors have cited simple, specific strategies to facilitate critical thinking in any situation. For simplicity's sake, these are summarized in Display 2–4. How many of these strategies have *you* used?

Critical Thinking Skills

Experts have identified a number of skills that must be mastered to think critically. These are listed starting on page 33, together with examples of how the skills are used in a nursing situation. Read through this list once, to get an idea of what we're talking about: After you've done this, there will be a brief discussion, and I'll be asking you to read the list again, asking yourself some questions.

Display 2–4	Strategies Enhancing Critical Thinking

Anticipate the questions others might ask (e.g., "What will my instructor want to know?" or "What will the doctor want to know?"). *Rationale.* This helps identify a wider scope of questions that need to be answered to gain relevant information.

Ask "why?" (determine underlying reasons). *Rationale.* To fully understand something, you must know *what* it is and *why* it's so. There's a saying, "She who knows what and how is likely to get a good job. She who knows *why*, is likely to be her boss."

Ask "what else" questions. For example, change "Have I done everything?" to "What else do I have to do?" *Rationale.* "What else" questions push you to look further and be more complete.

Ask "what if" questions like, "What if the worst happens?" or "What if we try...?" *Rationale.* This helps you be proactive, instead of reactive. It enhances your creativity and helps you put things in perspective.

Paraphrase in your own words. *Rationale.* Paraphrasing helps you understand information using a familiar language (your own).

Compare and contrast. *Rationale.* This forces you to look closely at the *parts* of something as well as the *whole,* helping you get more familiar with both things you're comparing. For example, If I asked you to compare two different kinds of apples, you'd have to *look closely at both of them.* As a result of comparing them, you'd also be more likely to know and *remember* each type of apple better.

Organize and reorganize information. *Rationale.* Organizing information helps you see certain patterns, but it may make you *miss* others; reorganizing information helps you see some of those *other* patterns. For example, compare the group of numbers in *a* below with the group of numbers listed in *b* and *c* below (each group contains the same numbers, organized differently). What patterns do you see?

a. 3634563   b. 34343   566   c. 333   44   566

Look for flaws in your thinking. Ask questions like, "What's missing?" and "How could this be made better?" *Rationale.* If you don't go looking for flaws, you'll be unlikely to find them. Once you've found them, you can make corrections early.

Ask someone else to look for flaws in your thinking. *Rationale.* This offers a "fresh eye" for evaluation, and may bring new ideas and perspectives.

Develop "good habits of inquiry" (habits that aid in the search for the truth, such as keeping an open mind, verifying information, and taking enough time). *Rationale.* Forming good habits helps make critical thinking more automatic.

Revisit information. *Rationale.* When you come back and look at something after a period of time, you'll be likely to view it differently: The passage of time not only helps you be more objective, but also you'll be likely to bring new knowledge you've gained to assessing the situation.

| Display 2–4 | Strategies Enhancing Critical Thinking (*Continued*) |

Replace the phrases "I don't know" or "I'm not sure" with "I need to find out." *Rationale.* This demonstrates you have the confidence and ability to find answers and mobilizes you to locate resources.

Turn errors into learning opportunities. *Rationale.* We all make mistakes—they're stepping stones to maturity and new ideas.

Share your mistakes—they're VALUABLE. *Rationale.* Sharing your mistakes helps others avoid making the same mistake, and may identify a common misconception or problem that needs to be rectified.

Adapted from Alfaro-LeFevre, R. (1994). Teaching nurses critical thinking. © *Academy of Medical-Surgical News, 3* (2), 4.

- **Identifying assumptions:** Recognizing when something is presented as fact, without proof. *Example.* Someone reports to you that a surgical patient is having incisional pain. You ask, "What is the pain like?" and the person responds, "I didn't ask, but he had surgery this morning, so it's got to be his incision." In fact, the pain could be related to any number of problems, ranging from a severe headache to a heart attack.
- **Identifying an organized approach to discovery:** Choosing a systematic approach that enhances ability to collect all the relevant data. *Example.* Performing a physical exam using a head-to-toe approach (carefully examining the head, then the neck, then the trunk and arms, and so on, down to the toes).
- **Checking accuracy and reliability of data:** Verifying information to be sure it's factual. *Example.* Double-checking an infant's weight when it's significantly different from the previous weight measurements.
- **Distinguishing relevant from irrelevant:** Deciding what information is pertinent to the situation at hand. *Example.* Identifying the fact that someone's stepfather died of a heart attack as being irrelevant to the person's *physical* risk factors for a heart attack, but relevant to the persons's *emotional* risk factors for a heart attack (the fear may cause cardiac stress).
- **Recognizing inconsistencies:** Realizing when there are contradictions within the presented information. *Example.* Noting that a child's injuries were unlikely to have happened in the way the parents describe.
- **Distinguishing normal from abnormal and identifying cues (pieces of information that prompt you to suspect a problem):** *Example.* Recognizing that a normally slightly wheezy asthmatic is now wheezing more than usual.
- **Clustering related information:** Putting together pieces of data that seem as though they should go together, in order to get an idea of pat-

terns of how things are (or aren't) working. *Example.* Putting together complaints of *poor appetite* and *difficulty preparing meals because of depression.*

- **Identifying patterns:** Interpreting what patterns are suggested by the information you've clustered together. *Example.* Considering the information above, and deciding that the cues represent a pattern of nutritional problems.
- **Identifying missing information:** Recognizing what pieces of information (data) are missing, and finding the missing pieces. *Example.* Questioning the person above about food intake or recent weight change.
- **Drawing valid conclusions (supporting conclusions with evidence):** Making deductions that follow logically. *Example.* In the above case, deciding that if the person has a recent weight loss, and says he's eaten only soup because he's too depressed to think about meals, an appropriate nursing diagnosis might be *Altered nutrition: less than body requirements related to depression and loss of appetite as evidenced by statements of poor appetite, difficulty preparing meals because of depression, and 10-pound weight loss.*
- **Considering several different conclusions:** Making sure all other likely conclusions were ruled out. *Example.* Considering whether the weight loss above could be a sign of a more severe problem, such as *cancer,* or some other problem that should be evaluated by a physician.
- **Identifying underlying cause and setting priorities:** Differentiating between problems needing immediate attention or subsequent action. *Example.* Identifying depression as a causative factor for the nutritional problem above, and deciding one of the first actions should be consulting an expert (advanced practice nurse, physician, psychologist) to evaluate the depression. Could it be that an antidepressant is required?
- **Determining realistic goals:** Deciding what needs to be accomplished, and by when it should be accomplished. *Example. By the end of 2 weeks, the person will gain 2 pounds.*
- **Developing a comprehensive plan:** Predicting responses, weighing risks and benefits, reducing risks, and determining interventions (actions). *Example.* Anticipating that the person might still not eat, even with meals provided, and asking a family member to visit at least every other day to check on him. Anticipating that the person above may regress and become overly dependent, and deciding that the benefits of getting him nutritionally stable outweigh that risk.
- **Evaluating and correcting our thinking:** Double-checking ourselves to make sure we've correctly accomplished the above skills, and making any required changes. *Example.* Realizing we were unsure about the reliability of the above person's family and double-checking to be sure the family is visiting every other day.

Did you find yourself noticing that some of the skills are things you already do without realizing it? Are you wondering, "What's the point of addressing skills that seem like they should be automatic?" The point is, you may do these automatically in familiar situations, but if you're *unaware* of what you're doing, it will be more difficult to transfer these skills to *unfamiliar* situations. A key point to realize is that *critical thinking is contextual* (it happens within a set of circumstances for a specific purpose). These skills require job-specific *knowledge,* and must be mastered *within the context* that you're working. As beginning nurses, with limited knowledge, you'll have to rely heavily on resources (e.g., textbooks, nurse experts) to help you apply what you know about critical thinking to specific nursing situations.

In Chapter 5, you'll have the opportunity to practice critical thinking skills in nursing situations. For now, I'd like you to connect with *what you know* and identify *what you want to learn* by re-reading the bold print in the skills (pp. 33–34), and asking yourself two questions as you consider each one:

1. How often do I apply this skill in every-day situations?
2. Would I know how to do this in a specific nursing situation?

Summary

By now, you should have an idea of factors that influence your ability to think critically, and have identified strategies that help you improve your thinking. To solidify your knowledge of this chapter, review the Key Points on the next page, and then complete the end-of-chapter exercises. Once you've done that, you'll be ready to go on to the next chapter, which addresses critical thinking specific to nursing.

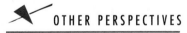

OTHER PERSPECTIVES

Motivation is what gets you started. Habit is what keeps you going.

Jim Ryun.

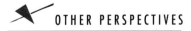

OTHER PERSPECTIVES

Remember the other 3 R's: Respect for yourself, respect for others, responsibility for your actions.

Brown, Life's Little Instruction Book, Vol. II.

KEY POINTS

▶ Chapter 1 focused on *what* critical thinking is and *why* it's important. This chapter focuses on *how* to think critically.

▶ Our ability to think well varies, depending on personal factors, and circumstances that might be evident at the time. Table 2–1 on page 21 lists factors enhancing and impeding critical thinking.

▶ Page 24 addresses common habits creating barriers to critical thinking (mine-is-better, choosing-only-one, face-saving, resistance to change, conformity, stereotyping, and self-deception).

▶ Steven Covey offers seven habits that can enhance critical thinking by helping us build positive interpersonal relationships (see Display 2–1 on page 26).

▶ Being aware of habits and factors influencing critical thinking helps us identify strategies that promote critical thinking.

▶ Critical thinking requires us to develop strategies that help us communicate effectively. Display 2–2 on page 27 provides communication techniques that can enhance critical thinking.

▶ There are eight key questions you need to ask to help you determine your approach to critical thinking in any situation. These are summarized in Display 2–3 on page 29.

▶ Logic provides a foundation for critical thinking. It's the safest and most reliable strategy for problem-solving.

▶ Using intuition as a guide to look for evidence is an effective strategy for critical thinking. *However,* before you act on intuition alone—before you act on gut feelings that aren't supported by evidence—be sure your actions won't cause harm.

▶ Trial-and-error, or trying several solutions until one that works is found, is a risky but sometimes necessary approach to problem-solving. It should be used only when there's plenty of room for error, when the problem can be monitored closely, and when the solutions have been logically thought through.

▶ To improve your ability to think critically, remember to ask questions like, "What's the big picture here?" "What's the small picture here?" "Am I considering both the parts and the whole?" and "Am I paying attention to details?"

▶ Display 2–4 on page 32 summarizes some simple but effective critical thinking strategies.

▶ Pages 33–34 list skills that must be mastered to think critically together with examples of how the skills are used in a nursing situation.

End-of-Chapter Exercises

Instructions:

Limit responses to 2–5 sentences.

Example responses for these exercises can be found in the *Response Key,* which begins on page 136.

1. How does knowing your preferred learning style influence your ability to think critically?

2. What would you say is your preferred learning style? If you don't know, study pages 147–149.

3. Complete the pre-chapter self-test, which has been reproduced below.

    a. Address five factors that influence critical thinking and explain how or why each one is influential.

    b. Explain how human habits can influence critical thinking ability.

    c. Give five practical strategies that can enhance critical thinking, and explain why the strategies work.

    d. Explain why developing effective interpersonal and communication skills is essential to critical thinking.

    e. Identify the roles of logic, intuition, and trial-and-error in critical thinking.

    f. Discuss at least five critical thinking skills you'd like to improve, and how you intend to improve them.

CRITICAL MOMENTS

When you're trying to understand, explain, or remember something, try drawing pictures, diagrams, or graphs. Our brains usually do better with pictures than words. For example, which of the ways of expressing percentages provided below is easiest for you to *understand?*

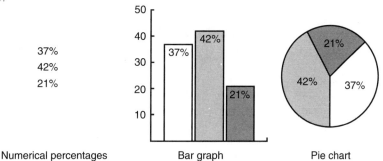

Numerical percentages   Bar graph   Pie chart

CRITICAL MOMENTS

On Mastery

Knowing you've mastered information or tasks is a strong motivator for doing *more.* Every so often, write down your recent accomplishments and see what else you'd like *to do.*

Critical Thinking in Nursing: An Overview

This chapter at a glance . . . .

Why Read This Chapter?

PRE-CHAPTER SELF-TEST

Read the objectives listed below and decide whether you can readily achieve each one. If you can, skip this chapter, and go on to Chapter 4. Don't be concerned if you can't meet any of the objectives at this time. We'll come back to this self-test at the end of the chapter, so you'll get a second chance.

O B J E C T I V E S

1. Discuss how critical thinking in nursing is similar to and different from critical thinking in any situation.

2. Define critical thinking in nursing and give four nursing situations when critical thinking is required.

3. Name two major goals of nursing and discuss their implications for critical thinking.

4. Explain how your level of knowledge and expertise (novice or expert) influences your ability to think critically.

5. Discuss the relationship of the nursing process to critical thinking.

6. Describe clinical judgment as addressed by Tanner (1983) and del Bueno (1994).

7. Identify a system for determining immediate priorities.

8. Explain how national and facility standards and guidelines are used as aids to decision-making.

9. Describe five key strategies for developing clinical judgment.

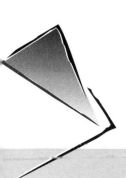

ABSTRACT

This chapter, the first of two focusing on how to improve your ability to think critically in relation to nursing's concerns, begins by pointing out that there are six categories of critical thinking that are integral to nursing. These categories are: clinical judgment (clinical reasoning), moral and ethical reasoning, nursing research, teaching others, teaching ourselves, and test-taking. The goals of nursing and their implications for critical thinking are addressed. To help you set realistic goals, differences in novice and expert thinking are presented. Emphasis is given to using the nursing process as a tool to promote critical thinking. Finally, this chapter answers the question, "What is clinical judgment, and how do you develop it?"

What Is Critical Thinking in Nursing?

At the big-picture level, critical thinking in nursing is similar to critical thinking in any situation. For example, critical thinking in nursing requires developing characteristics of critical thinkers (see page 10), it's influenced by the factors we addressed in Chapter 2, and it involves mastering critical thinking skills (see page 31). However, we need to keep two things in mind:

1. We as nurses must develop a *professional level* of critical thinking ability and performance that's different from that expected of others.
2. Critical thinking is contextual. It changes, depending on circumstances, even within nursing: For example, critical thinking in the clinical setting (real situations) differs from critical thinking in the classroom (simulated situations).

This section (Chapters 3 and 4) focuses on how to improve your ability to think critically in relation to nursing's major concerns. It addresses six categories of critical thinking that are integral to nursing, but require slightly different approaches. These categories are: clinical judgment (clinical reasoning), moral and ethical reasoning, nursing research, teaching others, teaching ourselves, and test-taking.

To keep the length of the chapters short enough to make the end-of-chapter exercises manageable—to avoid asking you to do too much at one time—content is divided into two chapters. This chapter provides an overview of critical thinking in nursing and examines how to develop clinical judgment (clinical reasoning skills). Chapter 4 addresses moral and ethical reasoning, nursing research, teaching ourselves, teaching others, and test-taking.

An Applied Definition of Critical Thinking

To understand the *specifics* of nursing's critical thinking, let's start by reviewing the applied definition from Chapter 1.

Critical thinking in nursing:

- Entails purposeful, goal-directed thinking.
- Aims to make judgments based on evidence (fact) rather than conjecture (guesswork).
- Is based on principles of science and scientific method (e.g., maintaining a questioning attitude, following an organized approach to discovery, and making sure information is reliable).
- Requires strategies that maximize *human potential* (e.g., tapping on individual strengths) and compensate for problems caused by *human nature* (e.g., the powerful influence of personal perceptions, values, and beliefs).

Some examples of when critical thinking is essential in nursing are when trying to:

- Get a better understanding of something or someone.
- Identify actual and potential problems.
- Make decisions about an action plan.
- Reduce risks of getting undesirable results.
- Increase the likelihood of achieving beneficial results.
- Find ways to improve (even when no problems exist).

Goals of Nursing and Their Implications

To understand nursing's critical thinking, it's essential to consider the questions, "What are the goals of nursing (what do nurses aim to do)?" and "What are the implications of these goals?"

Broadly speaking, nurses seek to accomplish two major goals in a humanistic, cost-effective, and timely fashion:

1. To help people avoid illness and its complications.
2. To help people gain an optimum level of independence and sense of well-being, regardless of health state (in cases of terminal illness, the goal of achieving a peaceful death is also appropriate).

So, what are the implications of these goals? Three major implications follow:

1. Because the conclusions and decisions we as nurses make *affect people's lives,* our thinking must be guided by sound reasoning—precise, disciplined thinking that promotes accuracy and depth of data collection, and seeks to clearly identify the issues at hand.

2. Because we're committed to giving humanistic care, we must seek to help people within the context of *their* value systems—value systems that may be different from our own. We need to be aware of the *moral* and *ethical dimensions* of our thinking: We face situations that require making decisions about when to withhold judgment and when to speak up and say, "No, that's wrong."

3. Because we're committed to achieving these goals in a cost-effective, timely fashion, we must constantly seek to improve both our personal ability to give nursing care *and* the overall efficiency of health care delivery.

Having made the above points, let's continue to look more closely at nursing's critical thinking, beginning with a discussion of how novice thinking differs from that of the expert. If we're aware of the differences, we'll be better able to set realistic goals for developing critical thinking specific to nursing.

Novice Thinking Versus Expert Thinking

Consider the following scenario:

Scenario One ■ A young man, riding his bicycle in the park, is hit by a car. Thrown 60 feet, he lies motionless. Within minutes, two park rangers arrive. They put on latex gloves, and begin to assess his injuries. An ambulance pulls up and one ranger yells, "We'll need intubation equipment!" A woman, out for a walk, looks on from a distance. A second woman, biking, comes upon the scene. Here's how the conversation goes:

First woman: This is terrible. I wish the ambulance had gotten here sooner.

Biking woman: Oh?

First woman: Yes. He was thrown at least 50 feet. If the ambulance had arrived sooner, they could have done more. I can't believe these two rangers didn't start resuscitation right away. They waited for this ambulance . . . they should have been breathing for him.

Biking woman: These rangers look like they know what they're doing. They would have started resuscitation if he needed it. This young man has been thrown so far, I'm sure they're concerned about spinal cord injuries. If they tilt his head back to start respirations, they risk severing his spinal cord—they don't want to do that unless it's absolutely necessary.

The above is a true story. I was the biking woman. As I talked more with the first woman, I learned she was a student nurse. She thanked me for pointing out something she hadn't thought about. After it was all over, I realized our conversation demonstrated a common difference between expert and novice thinking: The student nurse felt a need to *act* immediately. As an experienced nurse, I remembered the importance of *assessing* before acting.

We're all novices at one time or another. We all know what it's like to be new at something, and watch an experienced professional and wonder,

"Will *I* ever know this much?" And, almost always, with time and commitment, we soon find ourselves helping someone *else* who looks at *us,* and thinks, "Will *I* ever know this much?"

To help you gain insight into novice thinking and expert thinking, study Table 3–1, which compares the two: If you're a novice, determine some things you can do to enhance your ability to think critically; if you're an expert, decide how you can help a novice. Once you've done

Table 3–1

NOVICE NURSE THINKING COMPARED WITH EXPERT NURSE THINKING

The depth and breadth of expert knowledge, largely gained from opportunities to apply theory *in real situations,* greatly enhance critical thinking ability.

Novice Nurses	Expert Nurses
Knowledge is organized as separate facts. Must rely heavily on resources (texts, notes, preceptors). Lack knowledge gained from actually *doing* (e.g., listening to breath sounds).	Knowledge is highly organized and structured, making recall of information easier. Have a large storehouse of experiential knowledge (e.g., what abnormal breath sounds sound like, what subtle changes look like).
Focus so much on *actions,* they tend to forget to *assess* before acting.	*Assess* and think things through before *acting.*
Need clear-cut rules.	Know when to bend the rules.
Are often hampered by unawareness of resources.	Are aware of resources and how to use them.
Are often hindered by anxiety and lack of self-confidence.	Are usually more self-confident, less anxious, and therefore more focused.
Must be able to rely on step-by-step procedures. Tend to focus more on *procedures* than the *patient response* to the procedure.	Know when it's safe to skip steps or do two steps together. Are able to focus on both the parts (the procedures) and the whole (the patient response).
Become uncomfortable if patient needs preclude performing procedures exactly as they were learned.	Comfortable with rethinking procedure if patient needs require modification of the procedure.
Have limited knowledge of suspected problems; therefore, they question and collect data more superficially.	Have a better idea of suspected problems, allowing them to question more deeply, and collect more relevant and in-depth data.
Tend to follow standards and policies by rote.	Analyze standards and policies, looking for ways to improve them.
Learn more readily when matched with a supportive, knowledgeable preceptor or mentor.	Are challenged by novices' questions, clarifying their own thinking when teaching novices.

that, let's go on to consider the nursing process: The method nurses use to promote precise, disciplined thinking.

Nursing Process

Just as the problem-solving method provides a basis for precise, disciplined thinking in every-day situations, the nursing process provides the basis for critical thinking in nursing. Like the problem-solving method, the nursing process consists of five steps—*Assessment, Diagnosis, Planning, Implementation, and Evaluation (ADPIE)*—designed to expedite problem identification and treatment.

When we first began using the nursing process over 30 years ago, the steps were rather vague, and lacked details about how each step should be completed. It was more problem oriented than improvement oriented. However, nurses now recognize the need to provide detailed guidelines for using the nursing process in such a way that it enhances critical thinking.

Display 3–1	The Nursing Process As a Tool for Critical Thinking

- **Assessment.** Continuous, deliberate data collection designed to provide the information required to:
  - Predict, detect, prevent, control, or eliminate health problems.
  - Identify ways of helping people obtain optimum wellness and independence.
- **Diagnosis.** The process of analyzing data, putting related information together, drawing conclusions, and identifying:
  - Actual and potential health problems.
  - Underlying causes of the health problems.
  - Resources and strenghts.
  - Health states that are satisfactory, but could be improved.
- **Planning.** Determination of *specific* goals (desired outcomes) and interventions. The interventions are designed to:
  - Achieve the desired outcomes in a timely fashion.
  - Detect and prevent new health problems.
  - Promote optimum wellness and independence.
- **Implementation.** Putting the plan into action by:
  - Assessing readiness to act.
  - Acting, then reassessing to determine initial responses.
  - Making immediaate changes as needed.
  - Keeping records to monitor progress.
- **Evaluation.** Determining whether the expected outcomes have been met by comparing the patient's current assessment data with the outcomes recorded during *Planning*; modifying or terminating the plan as appropriate; planning for ongoing continuous assessment and improvement.

If you aren't familiar with the nursing process steps, study Display 3–1, which summarizes the key activities of each step, as used today to promote critical thinking. These are the steps that, when followed consistently, help you develop habits that promote critical thinking in nursing. Keep in mind that the accuracy of each step depends on the *accuracy of the preceding step*. For example, if the information you gathered during *Assessment* is inaccurate or incomplete, then *all the following steps* are likely to be inaccurate; if you've diagnosed the problems incorrectly, or missed problems altogether during *Diagnosis,* then *Planning, Implementation,* and *Evaluation* are likely to be inaccurate.

In Chapter 5, you'll have opportunities to practice various skills used in the nursing process. For now, consider Figure 3–1, which compares how the nursing process might be used by a nurse who thinks critically with how it might be used by a nurse who doesn't think critically.

Clinical Judgment (Clinical Reasoning)

The terms *clinical judgment, clinical reasoning,* and *critical thinking* are often used interchangeably. For example, you might hear, "Nursing requires effective clinical judgment" or "Nursing requires effective clinical

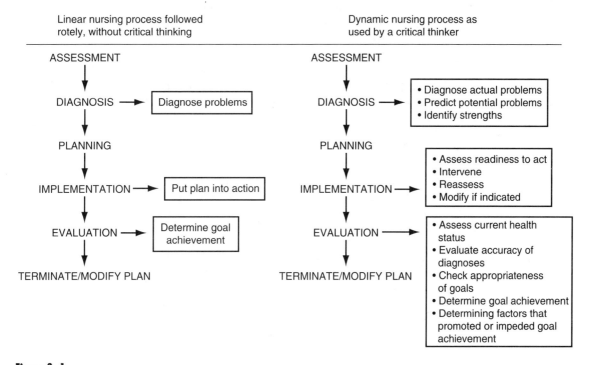

Figure 3–1
How a non–critical thinker might use the nursing process compared with how a critical thinker might use the nursing process, focusing on the diagnosis, implementation, and evaluation stages.

reasoning" or "Nursing requires critical thinking." We'll define clinical judgment as *critical thinking in the clinical area*.

Let's take a look at clinical judgment: What is it, and how do you develop it?

Developing clinical judgment is perhaps one of the most important and challenging aspects of becoming a nurse. It's important because the clinical area is where we first learn to think like a nurse in real client-nurse interactions. It's challenging because you usually have less time to make decisions, and it's often fraught with more anxiety and risks than other situations. For students, clinical reasoning is particularly challenging because it requires an ability to *recall facts, put them together into a meaningful whole, and apply the information to new situations*. For example: You note that someone is pale, sweaty, and has a rapid pulse. To be an effective nurse, you need to be able to recall that these are possible symptoms of shock, and that an immediate priority is to take a complete set of vital signs to further evaluate the patient's condition.

If you've developed general critical thinking skills, you'll find that once you're consistently in the clinical area, you'll begin to develop clinical reasoning skills quite quickly. The challenge of being in dynamic, real situations is a strong motivator for learning. The powerful effect of personal experience helps you remember information and be able to recall it to make judgments in *different* situations.

So, we know that developing clinical judgment is important and challenging. But what does it involve?

According to Tanner (1983), who has studied clinical judgment since the 1970's, clinical judgment usually involves making a series of decisions that includes deciding:

- What to observe.
- What data suggest.
- What actions to take.

Del Bueno (1994) has studied the clinical judgment of new graduates in both the United States and Canada. She adds to our understanding of clinical judgment by stating that to practice safely, new graduates must be able to:

- Identify essential data indicative of an acute change in health status.
- Differentiate between problems needing immediate attention and those requiring subsequent action.
- Initiate independent and collaborative actions to correct or minimize risks to health.
- Know why these actions are appropriate.

Nursing Diagnoses Versus Collaborative Problems

An integral part of developing clinical judgment is learning when to develop an independent plan (treat nursing diagnoses) and when to collaborate (seek medical consultation for potential medical problems). Let's consider the questions, "What's the difference between a nursing diagnosis and a collaborative problem?" "Which is more important?" and "How do I know which of these should be treated first?"

Nursing Diagnoses

In the literature and among nurses there's been much discussion about what *is* and what *isn't* a nursing diagnosis. Most often, nursing diagnoses are described in two ways:

1. **Nursing diagnoses are human responses** (how people respond to health problems or changes in life).* For example, a mother who's just broken her leg may be having difficulty with dealing with the many demands of her family, and might respond by demonstrating the nursing diagnosis of *Ineffective Individual Coping.*
2. **Nursing diagnoses are problems for which nurses are accountable for diagnosing and treating independently.** For example, if a patient is to be discharged home with a colostomy, it's nursing's responsibility to identify learning needs and provide the required instruction. In this case, an appropriate nursing diagnosis would be *Knowledge Deficit: Colostomy Care.*

Nursing diagnoses are best identified by using a nursing model to collect and organize data. Tables 3–2 and 3–3 show two commonly used nursing models. Chapter 5 (page 105) provides an example of an assessment tool that helps you collect data according to a nursing model.

In the hospital setting, you might encounter only a few nursing diag-

---

Table 3–2

FUNCTIONAL HEALTH PATTERNS (GORDON, 1987)

Health perception/health management pattern: Perception of health and well-being, knowledge of and adherence to regimens promoting health.
Nutritional-metabolic pattern: Usual food and fluid intake; height, weight, age.
Elimination pattern: Usual bowel and bladder elimination patterns.
Activity-rest pattern: Usual activity and exercise tolerance. Usual hours of exercise and rest.
Cognitive-perception pattern: Ability to use all senses to perceive environment. Usual way of perceiving environment.
Self-perception/self-concept pattern: Perception of capabilities and self-worth.
Role-relationship pattern: Usual responsibilities and ways of relating to others.
Sexuality-reproductive pattern: Knowledge and perception of sex and reproduction.
Coping–stress tolerance pattern: Ability to manage and tolerate stress.
Value-belief pattern: Values, beliefs, and goals in life. Spiritual practices.

---

*The official definition of nursing diagnosis published by the North American Nursing Diagnosis Association (NANDA) can be found in the glossary.

Table 3-3

HUMAN RESPONSE PATTERNS

Exchanging

Cardiac	Cerebral
Peripheral	Skin integrity
Oxygenation	Physical regulation
Nutrition	Elimination

Communicating

Read/write/understand English, other languages, impaired speech, other forms of communication

Relating

Relationships	Socialization

Valuing

Religious preference, important religious practices, spiritual concerns, cultural orientation, cultural practices

Choosing

Coping	Participation in health regimen
Judgment	

Moving

Activity	Rest
Recreation	Environmental maintenance
Health maintenance	Self-care
Meaningfulness	Sensory perception

Perceiving

Self-concept	Meaningfulness
Sensory perception	

Knowing

Current health problems	Health history
Current medications	Risk factors
Readiness to learn	Mental status
Memory	

Feeling

Pain/discomfort associated/aggravating/alleviating factors
Emotional integrity/status

From Iyer, P.W., Taptich, B.J., and Bernocchi-Losey, D. (1991). *Nursing process and nursing diagnosis* (2nd ed., p. 51). Philadelphia: W.B. Saunders Co.

noses being formally addressed. The reason for this is that short hospital stays and cost containment efforts cause hospitals to adopt strict policies for setting priorities: They usually address *only* those problems that must be resolved in order for people to be discharged from the hospital and care for themselves at home. For example, suppose you have someone with two nursing diagnoses, one related to family problems (e.g., *Altered Family Processes*) and the other related to knowledge that must be gained before discharge (e.g., *Knowledge Deficit: Wound Care*). Which of these two diagnoses do you think is given higher priority? If you thought

Knowledge Deficit: Wound Care, you're correct. Depending on the severity of the problem, *Altered Family Processes* is likely to be dealt with by advising the family of community resources, or by referring the problem to the social services or home care department.

In community and long-term care settings, you'll see more nursing diagnoses being addressed because there is more time and more family involvement, and nursing care focuses more on optimum wellness than simply curing disease.

Display 3–2 provides the list of nursing diagnoses accepted for clinical testing by the North American Nursing Diagnosis Association (NANDA). Because the listed diagnoses are in various stages of development, and because some are controversial, I recommend that if you're a beginner, ask your instructor which diagnoses you should learn first.

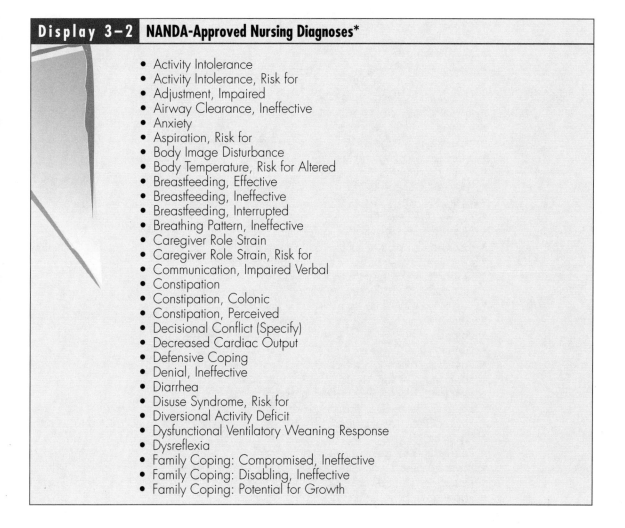

Display 3–2	NANDA-Approved Nursing Diagnoses*

- Activity Intolerance
- Activity Intolerance, Risk for
- Adjustment, Impaired
- Airway Clearance, Ineffective
- Anxiety
- Aspiration, Risk for
- Body Image Disturbance
- Body Temperature, Risk for Altered
- Breastfeeding, Effective
- Breastfeeding, Ineffective
- Breastfeeding, Interrupted
- Breathing Pattern, Ineffective
- Caregiver Role Strain
- Caregiver Role Strain, Risk for
- Communication, Impaired Verbal
- Constipation
- Constipation, Colonic
- Constipation, Perceived
- Decisional Conflict (Specify)
- Decreased Cardiac Output
- Defensive Coping
- Denial, Ineffective
- Diarrhea
- Disuse Syndrome, Risk for
- Diversional Activity Deficit
- Dysfunctional Ventilatory Weaning Response
- Dysreflexia
- Family Coping: Compromised, Ineffective
- Family Coping: Disabling, Ineffective
- Family Coping: Potential for Growth

Display 3–2	NANDA-Approved Nursing Diagnoses* (*continued*)

- Family Processes, Altered
- Fatigue
- Fear
- Fluid Volume Deficit
- Fluid Volume Deficit, Risk for
- Fluid Volume Excess
- Gas Exchange, Impaired
- Grieving, Anticipatory
- Grieving, Dysfunctional
- Growth and Development, Altered
- Health Maintenance, Altered
- Health Seeking Behaviors (Specify)
- Home Maintenance Management, Impaired
- Hopelessness
- Hyperthermia
- Hypothermia
- Incontinence, Bowel
- Incontinence, Functional
- Incontinence, Reflex
- Incontinence, Stress
- Incontinence, Total
- Incontinence, Urge
- Individual Coping, Ineffective
- Infant Feeding Pattern, Ineffective
- Infection, Risk for
- Injury, Risk for
- Knowledge Deficit (Specify)
- Management of Therapeutic Regimen (Individuals), Ineffective
- Noncompliance (Specify)
- Nutrition: Less Than Body Requirements, Altered
- Nutrition: More Than Body Requirements, Altered
- Nutrition: Potential for More Than Body Requirements, Altered
- Oral Mucous Membrane, Altered
- Pain
- Pain, Chronic
- Parental Role Conflict
- Parenting, Altered
- Parenting, Risk for Altered
- Peripheral Neurovascular Dysfunction, Risk for
- Personal Identity Disturbance
- Physical Mobility, Impaired
- Poisoning, Risk for
- Post-Trauma Response
- Powerlessness
- Protection, Altered
- Rape-Trauma Syndrome

| Display 3-2 | **NANDA-Approved Nursing Diagnoses*** (*continued*) |

- Rape-Trauma Syndrome: Compound Reaction
- Rape-Trauma Syndrome: Silent Reaction
- Relocation Stress Syndrome
- Role Performance, Altered
- Self Care Deficit
  - Bathing/Hygiene
  - Dressing/Grooming
  - Feeding
  - Toileting
- Self Esteem, Chronic Low
- Self Esteem, Situational Low
- Self Esteem Disturbance
- Sensory/Perceptual Alterations (Specify) (Visual, Auditory, Kinesthetic, Gustatory, Tactile, Olfactory)
- Self-Mutilation, Risk for
- Sexual Dysfunction
- Sexuality Patterns, Altered
- Skin Integrity, Impaired
- Skin Integrity, Risk for Impaired
- Sleep Pattern Disturbance
- Social Interaction, Impaired
- Social Isolation
- Spiritual Distress
- Suffocation, Risk for
- Sustain Spontaneous Ventilation, Inability to
- Swallowing, Impaired
- Thermoregulation, Ineffective
- Thought Processes, Altered
- Tissue Integrity, Impaired
- Tissue Perfusion, Altered (Specify Type) (Renal, Cerebral, Cardiopulmonary, Gastrointestinal, Peripheral)
- Trauma, Risk for
- Unilateral Neglect
- Urinary Elimination, Altered
- Urinary Retention
- Violence, Risk for: Self-Directed or Directed at Others

*Up-to-date listing of diagnoses accepted for clinical use. Diagnoses added in 1994 were accepted for *study*, not *clinical use*. North American Nursing Diagnosis Association (1992). NANDA Nursing Diagnoses: Definitions and Classification 1992–1993. Philadelphia: NANDA.

Collaborative Problems

Collaborative problems are so named because the approach to their treatment is *collaborative* (Carpenito, 1993). Usually a physician or medical protocols prescribe what must be done to manage the problem and (if necessary) what must be *avoided* to prevent aggravating the problem.

Once this information is obtained, the other health care professionals (nurses, physical therapists, speech therapists, etc.) can then identify independent actions that are *specific* to the person's individual needs. For instance, the physician might prescribe an anti-inflammatory medication and physical therapy. If so, then the nurse and physical therapist would tailor interventions to the patient's specific needs (e.g., the nurse would assess for history of gastrointestinal symptoms and ensure that all doses

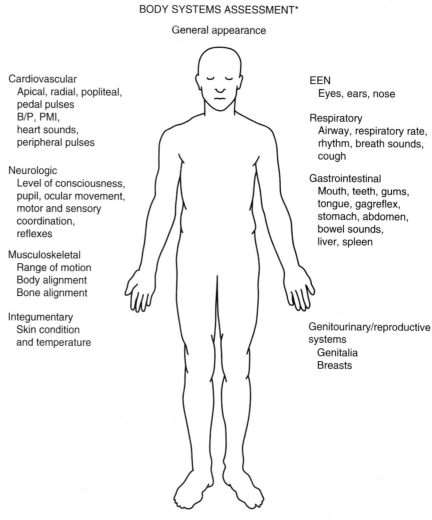

BODY SYSTEMS ASSESSMENT*

General appearance

Cardiovascular
Apical, radial, popliteal, pedal pulses
B/P, PMI, heart sounds, peripheral pulses

Neurologic
Level of consciousness, pupil, ocular movement, motor and sensory coordination, reflexes

Musculoskeletal
Range of motion
Body alignment
Bone alignment

Integumentary
Skin condition and temperature

EEN
Eyes, ears, nose

Respiratory
Airway, respiratory rate, rhythm, breath sounds, cough

Gastrointestinal
Mouth, teeth, gums, tongue, gagreflex, stomach, abdomen, bowel sounds, liver, spleen

Genitourinary/reproductive systems
Genitalia
Breasts

* Pain associated with any system should be recorded.

Figure 3–2
Body systems assessment.

were taken with food; the physical therapist would help the patient gradually increase movement, according to patient tolerance).

Collaborative problems usually involve problems with structure or function of organs or systems. For this reason, they're best identified by using a body system approach to organizing data (Fig. 3–2). In Chapter 5, you'll have opportunities to organize data according to body systems and according to a nursing model. For now, there are three things to remember:

1. Nursing models (see Tables 3–2 and 3–3, pages 47 and 48) help you identify nursing diagnoses.
2. Body system models help you identify data that the physician must be aware of.
3. You need to use *both* models to be sure you identify nursing diagnoses and collaborative problems.

An essential nursing role in relation to collaborative problems is that of predicting, preventing, detecting, and managing *potential complications*. Display 3–3 (next page) lists commonly encountered collaborative problems and related potential complications. These are all common problems that nurses must become familiar with before graduating from nursing school.

Deciding Which Are More Important

So the question still unanswered is: Which are more important, nursing diagnoses or collaborative problems? The answer is, they're *both* important, but you need to decide what you'll do *first*. You need to identify immediate priorities, and then go on to develop a plan for the other problems, which are important, but usually not quite as urgent.

Setting Immediate Priorities

Here's a suggestion to help you decide what to do first, when faced with nursing diagnoses and collaborative problems. Remember that frequently nursing diagnoses are human responses *to* medical problems. This means that in many cases, if the person didn't have the *medical* problem in the first place, he wouldn't have the *nursing diagnosis*, right? So it would be wise to assess the medical problems before going on to identify nursing diagnoses, correct? If you start by assessing signs and symptoms that might indicate a medical problem, and assessing responses to medical treatments already initiated, you can ensure that any required medical treatment is begun. Then you can go on to diagnose and treat nursing diagnoses. If you don't report signs and symptoms of suspected medical problems immediately, you may be delaying essential medical care. For these reasons, it's wise to take the following approach to set immediate priorities:

| Display 3-3 | **Common Collaborative Problems** |

Common medical diagnoses (in **bold**) and their potential complications

- **Angina/myocardial infarction**
  - Dysrhythmias
  - Congestive heart failure/pulmonary edema
  - Shock (cardiogenic, hypovolemic)
  - Infarction, infarction extension
  - Thrombi/emboli formation (e.g., pulmonary emboli, cerebrovascular accident)
  - Hypoxemia
  - Electrolyte imbalance
  - Acid-base imbalance
  - Pericarditis
  - Cardiac tamponade
  - Cardiac arrest
- **Asthma/chronic obstructive lung disease**
  - Hypoxemia
  - Acid-base/electrolyte imbalance
  - Respiratory failure
  - Cardiac failure
  - Infection
- **Diabetes**
  - Hyper/hypoglycemia
  - Delayed wound healing
  - Hypertension
  - Eye problems (retinal hemorrhage)
  - *See also* angina/myocardial infarction
- **Fractures**
  - Bleeding
  - Fracture displacement
  - Thrombus/embolus formation
  - Compromised circulation
  (pressure points, edema)
  - Nerve compression
  - Infection
  - *See also* skeletal traction/casts
- **Head trauma**
  - Increased intracranial pressure (secondary to bleeding or brain swelling)
  - Respiratory depression
  - Shock
  - Hyper/hypothermia
  - Coma
- **Hypertension**
  - Cerebrovascular accident
  - Transient ischemic attacks (TIA's)
  - Renal failure
  - Hypertensive crisis
  - *See also* angina/myocardial infarction
- **Pneumonia**
  - Respiratory failure
  - Sepsis/septic shock
- **Pulmonary embolus**
  - *See* angina/myocardial infarction
- **Renal failure**
  - Fluid overload
  - Hyperkalemia
  - Electrolyte/acid-base imbalance
  - Anemia
  - *See also* hypertension
- **Trauma**
  - *See* anesthesia/surgical or invasive procedures
- **Urinary tract infection**

Common treatment and diagnostic modalities (in **bold**) and their potential complications

- **Anesthesia/surgical or invasive procedures**
  - Bleeding/hypovolemia/shock
  - Respiratory depression/atelectasis
  - Urinary retention
  - Fluid/electrolyte imbalances
  - Thrombus/embolus formation
  - Paralytic ileus
  - Incisional complications (infection, poor healing, dehiscence/evisceration)
  - Sepsis/septic shock

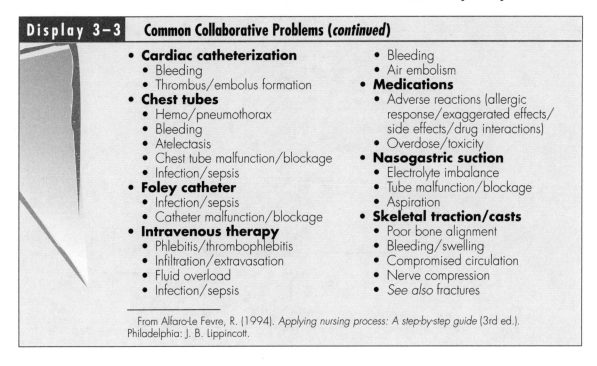

From Alfaro-Le Fevre, R. (1994). *Applying nursing process: A step-by-step guide* (3rd ed.). Philadelphia: J. B. Lippincott.

1. **First, identify signs and symptoms that might indicate a problem requiring medical treatment or not responding to medical treatment.** These are the problems you'll be treating *collaboratively*. You need to:

   - Make sure the physician is aware of the signs and symptoms.
   - Determine responses to medical treatments already initiated (is the patient responding as expected?).
   - Initiate urgent interventions as indicated by physician's orders, protocols, and other applicable plans of care.

2. **Second, study the data you've gathered by using a nursing model, and identify nursing diagnoses.** Your independent role as a nurse, helping the person adapt and deal with how the medical problems are affecting his life, is essential to developing a plan of care that promotes independence and well-being.

Scope of Practice Decisions

Another aspect of developing clinical judgment is learning to make decisions about what actions are within your scope of practice. In other words, how do you know when you're allowed to perform a nursing action? Several state boards of nursing have developed guides to help nurses make these types of decisions. Figure 3–3 shows one of these decision-making models adapted to help students decide whether an act is within their scope of practice.

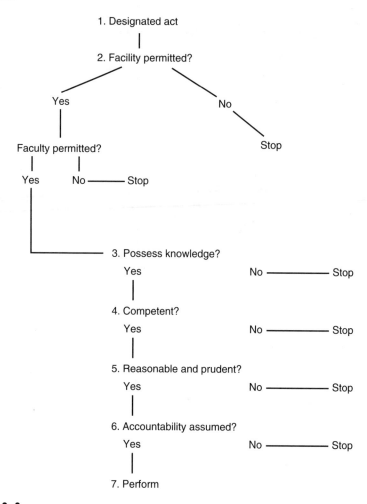

Figure 3–3
Model to aid student decision-making. (Adapted from Pennsylvania State Board of Nursing Decision Making Model.)

Decision-making and Nursing Standards and Guidelines

Decision-making in nursing is influenced by broad and specific standards and guidelines.

National standards for practice provide broad standards that address how nurses are expected to plan and deliver care (see Appendix E, standards of practice, on page 162). Each specialty organization (e.g., American Association of Critical-Care Nurses, Association of Rehabilitation Nurses, Association of Operating Room Nurses) has also developed its own standards for specialty practice.

Each facility has developed numerous specific standards and guidelines (standards of care, policies, protocols, procedures, care plans, and critical paths*) that are intended to aid decision-making in *specific* situations. The *Agency for Health Care Policy and Research* has also developed national practice guidelines for the care of some specific problems (see Display 3–4 on page 58).

There are two questions to raise when you're involved in making decisions about how to manage specific health problems:

1. Has this facility developed specific guidelines or policies for the care of this specific situation? For example, if you're caring for someone with a mastectomy, you need to ask, "Has this facility developed any type of guidelines for someone undergoing a mastectomy?"
2. Are there national practice guidelines relating to this particular problem?

If the answer to either of the above is yes, you must ask a third question:

3. To what degree do these standards apply to my specific patient's situation?

Facility and national guidelines are valuable tools to help you make care decisions. However, guidelines aren't meant to be followed *blindly*. An essential part of decision-making is using critical thinking to recognize when the situation at hand *differ*s from the guide. You must carefully *compare your patient's data with the information presented in the guideline,* and decide whether the guidelines are indeed applicable to your specific patient. For example, suppose you're caring for someone who just had prostate surgery, and the critical path for this problem states that on the second day, the patient will get out of bed twice. However, on the second day, you assess the man, and find he has chest discomfort. This finding is significant enough for you to question whether he should indeed get out of bed today: Could this man be suffering a complication such as myocardial infarction or pulmonary embolus? In this case, you need to report the symptoms, and keep the man in bed until he's been carefully evaluated by a physician.

How to Develop Effective Clinical Judgment

Developing clinical reasoning skills takes time. It also requires a commitment to study common health problems, seek out clinical experi-

---

*See Appendix D (page 155) for an example of critical path.

| Display 3–4 | **Agency for Health Care Policy and Research (AHCPR) Practice Guidelines*** |

Available as of 1994
- Acute low back problems
- Acute pain
- Benign prostatic hyperplasia
- Cataracts in adults
- Sickle cell disease
- Depression
- Early HIV infection
- Heart failure
- Management of cancer pain
- Otitis media
- Pressure ulcers in adults: prediction and prevention
- Quality determinants of mammography
- Treatment of pressure ulcers
- Urinary incontinence

Forthcoming after 1994
- Cancer screening
- Cardiac rehabilitation
- Colorectal cancer
- Post-stroke rehabilitation
- Screening for Alzheimer's disease
- Smoking cessation

*Guidelines are available in several formats: *Clinical Practice Guidelines* and *Quick Reference Guides for Clinicians* are intended for health care providers; *Consumer Versions*, also available in Spanish. are intended for patients and family members. For more information, contact: AHCPR Publications Clearinghouse, Box 8547, Silver Spring, MD 20907.

ences, and come prepared to the clinical setting. In the next chapters, you'll have opportunities to practice skills that are essential to critical thinking and developing clinical judgment. For now, review Display 3–5 on page 59, which answers the eight critical thinking questions from Chapter 2 in relation to clinical judgment. Once you've done that, consider the following strategies for developing effective clinical judgment.

Ten Strategies for Developing Effective Clinical Judgment

1. **Acquire a storehouse of facts as addressed below.** This is the information required to reason clinically: If you don't have these facts in long-term memory, keep references such as notes, texts, and pocket guides readily available.

   - **Learn terminology and concepts.** If you encounter words like *embolus, thrombus,* or *phlebitis,* and you don't know what they

| Display 3-5 | **Clinical Judgment (Clinical Reasoning): Key Questions** |

1. **What's the goal of my thinking?** To initiate a plan designed to expedite diagnosis and treatment of health problems, prevent potential health problems, and promote independence and a sense of well-being.

2. **What are the circumstances?** Circumstances vary: A major circumstance to consider is that you're dealing with real, rather than simulated, situations. Other circumstances to consider are: *Who's* involved (e.g., child, adult, group)? *What* are the problems? How urgent are the problems (e.g., life-threatening, chronic)? What are the factors influencing their presentation (e.g., When, where, and how did the problems develop)? What are the patient's values, beliefs, and cultural influences?

3. **What knowledge is required?** Knowledge required includes: problem-specific facts (e.g., how health problems usually present, how they're diagnosed, what causes them, what the associated potential complications are, and how these complications are prevented and managed); nursing process and related knowledge and skills (ethics, research, health assessment, communication, priority-setting, leadership); related sciences (anatomy, physiology, pathophysiology, pharmacology, chemistry, physics, psychology, sociology). You must also be clearly aware of the circumstances, as addressed in No. 2 above.

4. **How much room is there for error?** Room for error is usually minimal. However, it depends on the health state of the individual and the risks of the interventions. *Example:* In which of the following cases do you think you have more room for error?
   a. You're trying to decide whether to give a usually healthy child a one-time dose of acetaminophen (Tylenol) for heat rash without checking with the doctor.
   b. You have a child who's been sick for 3 days, you don't know what the illness is, and the mother wants to know if she should continue giving acetaminophen without checking with the doctor.
   If you thought *a*, you're correct. In situation *b*, the symptoms have continued for 3 days without a diagnosis. If you continue to give acetaminophen without checking with a physician, you might be masking symptoms of a problem requiring medical treatment.

5. **How much time do I have?** Time frame for decision-making depends on: (1) The urgency of the problems (e.g., there's less time in life-threatening situations, such as cardiac arrest). (2) The planned length of stay (e.g., if your patient will be hospitalized only for 2 days, key decisions need to be made *early*).

6. **What resources can help me?** Human resources include: clinical nurse educators, nursing faculty, preceptors, more experienced nurses, peers, librarians, and other health care professionals (pharmacists, nutritionists, physical therapists, physicians). The patient and family are also valuable resources (it isn't unusual for them to know their own problems best). Other resources include: texts, articles, other references, and computer data bases; national practice guidelines, facility documents (e.g., guidelines, policies, procedures, assessment forms).

| Display 3-5 | Clinical Judgment (Clinical Reasoning): Key Questions (*continued*) |

7. Whose perspectives *must* be considered? The most significant perspective to consider is that of the patient. Other important perspectives include those of the family and significant others, caregivers, and relevant third parties (e.g., insurers).

8. What's influencing my thinking? Thinking may be influenced by all the factors influencing critical thinking listed in Table 2-1 (page 21).

mean, you'll be unable to understand and learn. Comprehension begins with acquiring vocabulary. If you look up new terms and concepts *as you encounter them,* they'll soon become a part of your long-term memory. Learning the terms *in context* also helps you store information in related groups, rather than as isolated facts.

- **Become familiar with normal findings before being concerned with abnormal findings** (e.g., lab values, physical assessment findings, disease progression, growth and development): Once you know the *normals,* you'll readily recognize when you encounter information that is *outside the norm* (abnormal).
- **Always ask *why*.** Find out what theories or principles explain why *normal* findings occur, and why *abnormal* findings occur.
- **Learn problem-specific facts.** Clinical judgment is enhanced by your knowledge of such things as how problems usually present (their signs and symptoms), what usually causes them, and how they're usually managed. For instance, if you're going to take care of someone who has a medical diagnosis of *diabetes,* and a nursing diagnosis of *Ineffective Individual Coping,* you need to become familiar with the signs, symptoms, common causes, and common management of these two problems before caring for the person.

Experienced nurses often have problem-specific facts stored in long-term memory because they've repeatedly encountered similar situations. If you're a beginner, you need to rely on memorization and on keeping resources readily available. If you come to the clinical setting prepared, having studied the situations you'll be likely to encounter, and keep your resources close by, you'll improve your ability to demonstrate effective clinical judgment. You'll also begin to develop your own storehouse of problem-specific facts in long-term memory: What you learn through *experience* is remembered better than what you memorize. Display 3–6 provides questions you should ask to gain the facts you'll need to know to reason well in the clinical setting.

2. Use the nursing process as a guide to thinking. Always assess first to avoid jumping to conclusions, then go on to diagnose (identify the problem), plan, implement, and evaluate. Whenever possible, use principles of logic to promote making judgments based on *fact* rather

Display 3–6	Questions to Ask to Gain Problem-Specific Knowledge Before Taking Care of Someone in the Clinical Setting

1. What problems do I know or suspect my patient has?
2. What are the signs and symptoms of these problems?
3. What will I need to assess to determine the status of these signs and symptoms?
4. What are the usual causes of these problems?
5. What will I assess to determine the status of the *causes* of the problems?
6. How do these problems usually progress, and how are they managed?
7. How can these problems be prevented?
8. What could cause these problems to change, and in what way?
9. What are the signs and symptoms of potential complications of these problems, and how will I monitor for these signs and symptoms?
10. What other processes are likely to be seen along with these problems?
11. What medications and treatments are likely to be used, and why?
12. What medication-related or treatment-related problems might I encounter, how will I monitor to detect them, and how are they usually managed?
13. What cultural factors, values, or beliefs might have bearing on health practices in relation to these health problems?
14. What are the key things people need to know to manage these problems independently, and what will I do to ensure that this knowledge is gained?

than guesswork (see Using Logic, Intuition, and Trial-and-Error on page 30).

3. **Develop a systematic approach to assessment.** This will be addressed in greater depth in Chapter 5, where you'll have opportunities to practice using a systematic approach to discovery.

4. **Determine a system that helps you make decisions about what must be done now, and what can wait until later.**

   - **Be sure you identify the underlying causes of the problems:** Until you've identified the problem *and its cause,* you don't really understand the problem, or what has to be done immediately. For example, if you suspect someone's abdominal pain is caused by appendicitis, you know that a top priority in managing the situation is to consult a physician. If you treat the pain without medical evaluation, you'll mask symptoms, possibly delaying diagnosis of a serious problem.

   - **Always ask yourself, "Could any of these signs and symptoms be caused by an undetected problem with structure or function of an organ or system requiring medical treatment?"** If the answer is yes, an immediate priority, before going on to plan nursing care, is to notify a physician or your instructor or supervisor.

- **To make thinking more automatic, consistently use the same system to set immediate priorities.** An example of a system that's commonly used to set priorities is listed in Display 3–7.

5. **Never perform an action if you don't know why it's indicated, why it works (the rationale), and whether there are risks of harm.** When you understand why an action is specified, you know whether it's relevant and appropriate. When you know risks of harm, you can identify ways of reducing the risk. For example, if you're aware of the risks of introducing an air embolism into an IV line, you find ways to reduce that risk (e.g., taping connections together).

6. **Learn from your human resources (faculty, experts, classmates, other nurses), and when in doubt, get help from a qualified professional.** Your patients' rights to expedient care take precedence over your need to learn independently. Other professionals can help you decide whether you have time to look up your con-

---

Display 3–7 **A Common Approach to Identifying Immediate Priorities**

Treatment for first- and second-level priorities is usually initiated in rapid succession or simultaneously. *At times*, the order of priority might change, depending on the seriousness of the problem and relationship between the problems. For example, if abnormal lab values are life-threatening, they become a higher priority; if your patient is having trouble breathing because of acute pain, treating the pain might become the highest priority. It's important to consider the *relationship* between the problems: For example, if *Problem Y* causes *Problem Z*, *Problem Y* takes priority over *Problem Z*.

1. **First-level priority problems** (immediate priorities): Remember the ABC'S:
   - **A**irway problems
   - **B**reathing problems
   - **C**ardiac/circulation problems
   - **S**igns (vital **signs** concerns)
2. **Second-level priority problems** (immediate, after treatment for first-level problems is initiated)
   - **M**ental status change
   - **A**cute pain
   - **A**cute urinary elimination problems
   - **U**ntreated medical problems requiring immediate attention (e.g., a diabetic who hasn't had insulin)
   - **A**bnormal lab values
   - **R**isks of infection, safety, or security (for patient or for others)

Note: To help you remember the above, mnemonic MAA-U-AR provides the first letter of each of the second-level priority problems.

3. **Third-level priority problems** (later priorities)
   - Health problems that don't fit into the above categories (e.g., problems with lack of knowledge, activity, rest, family coping)

cerns in a reference. Let others know you'd like to learn more about various nursing situations. For example, you may care for someone who had a kidney stone removed, and learn just as much by asking classmates to tell you about the things they learned while taking care of *others* with different problems. Collaborating with classmates is a win-win situation: Asking questions like, "What did you look for?" "How did you know what to look for?" and "What was the biggest thing you learned?" will help your classmates clarify knowledge, and help you learn from being involved in real situations. **Note:** Keep in mind the ethics of discussing patient care: Don't use names or talk about patients in public places where others might overhear (e.g., cafeteria, elevators).

7. **Become familiar with facility standards (e.g., protocols, policies, procedures, critical paths) that relate to your patient's problems.** While these standards aren't meant to be followed *blindly*—their appropriateness to each specific patient must be determined—they've been developed by experts with good clinical judgment, and are intended to help you make decisions about key aspects of patient care.

8. **Practice manual skills (e.g., handling IV tubing, changing dressings).** If you aren't comfortable performing these skills, your ability to reason will be hampered by the stress of trying to master these technical procedures.

9. **Become familiar with the technology you'll use (e.g., IV pumps, computers, monitors).** These are intended to reduce some of the work of nursing.

10. **Remember the importance of *caring* (being willing to place great importance on the wants and needs of patients and their significant others).** More specifically, caring has been described by patients as *vigilance* (nurse attentiveness, highly skilled practice, basic care, nurturing, and going the extra mile); *mutuality* (relationships and behaviors generated among the nurse, patient, and family); and *healing* (life-saving behaviors and freeing the patient from anxiety and concerns) (Burfitt et al., 1993).

Summary

Critical thinking in nursing, guided by use of the nursing process, must be precise, disciplined thinking that promotes accuracy and depth of data collection, and seeks to clearly identify the issues at hand. This chapter presents an overview of critical thinking in nursing, and examines how to develop effective clinical judgment. To solidify your knowledge of this chapter, review the following key points, and complete the end-of-chapter exercises.

K E Y   P O I N T S

▶ This chapter provides an overview of critical thinking in nursing and examines how to develop clinical judgment (clinical reasoning skills).

▶ At the big-picture level, critical thinking in nursing is similar to critical thinking in any situation. For example, critical thinking in nursing requires developing attitudes of critical thinkers, it's influenced by the factors we addressed in Chapter 2, and it involves mastering critical thinking skills.

▶ We as nurses must develop a *professional level* of critical thinking ability and performance that's different from that expected of others. We must also keep in mind that critical thinking is contextual, changing with circumstances.

▶ Critical thinking in nursing: Entails purposeful, goal-directed thinking; aims to make judgments based on evidence (fact) rather than conjecture (guesswork); is based on principles of science and scientific method (e.g., maintaining a questioning attitude, following an organized approach to discovery, and making sure information is reliable); requires strategies that maximize *human potential* (e.g., using individual strengths), and compensate for problems caused by *human nature* (e.g., the powerful influence of personal perceptions, values, and beliefs).

▶ Some examples of when critical thinking is essential in nursing are when trying to: get a better understanding of something or someone; identify actual and potential problems; make decisions about an action plan; reduce risks of getting undesirable results; increase the likelihood of achieving beneficial results; find ways to improve (even when no problems exist).

▶ *Broadly speaking,* nurses seek to accomplish two major goals in a humanistic, cost-effective, and timely fashion: (1) To help people avoid illness and its complications. (2) To help people gain an optimum level of independence and sense of well-being, regardless of health state (in cases of terminal illness, the goal of achieving a peaceful death is also appropriate.)

▶ Because the conclusions and decisions we as nurses make *affect people's lives,* our thinking must be guided by sound reasoning—precise, disciplined thinking that promotes accuracy and depth of data collection, and seeks to clearly identify the issues at hand.

▶ We as nurses must be aware of the moral and ethical dimensions of our thinking, seeing to help people within the context of *their* value systems—value systems that may be different from our own.

▶ We must constantly seek to improve both our personal ability to give nursing care *and* the overall efficiency of health care delivery.

▶ How we think is greatly influenced by our knowledge and experience. Table 3–1 (page 43) compares novice and expert thinking.

▶ Just as the problem-solving method provides a basis for precise, disciplined critical thinking in everyday situations, the nursing process provides the basis for critical thinking in nursing. Like the problem-solving method, the nursing process consists of five steps—*Assessment, Diagnosis, Planning, Implementation, and Evaluation (ADPIE)*—designed to expedite problem identification and promote efficiency of health care delivery.

▶ The accuracy of each step of the nursing process depends on the *accuracy of the preceding step.* For example, if the information you gathered during *Assessment* is inaccurate or incomplete, then *all the following steps* are likely to be inaccurate; if you've diagnosed the problems incorrectly, or missed problems altogether during *Diagnosis,* then *Planning, Implementation,* and *Evaluation* are likely to be inaccurate.

▶ Display 3–1 (page 44) summarizes the key activities of each step of the nursing process as used today to promote critical thinking. Figure 3–1 (page 45) compares how the nursing process might be used by a nurse who thinks critically, to how it might be used by a nurse who *doesn't* think critically.

▶ The terms *clinical judgment, clinical reasoning,* and *critical thinking* are often used interchangeably. Developing clinical judgment is perhaps one of the most important and challenging aspects of becoming a nurse.

▶ According to Tanner (1983), clinical judgment usually involves making a series of decisions that includes deciding: what to observe, what data suggest, and what actions to take. Del Bueno (1994) adds to our understanding of clinical judgment by stating that to practice safely, new graduates must be able to: identify essential data indicative of an acute change in health status; initiate independent and collaborative actions to correct or minimize risks to patients' health; know why these actions are appropriate; and differentiate between problems needing immediate attention and those requiring subsequent action.

▶ Clinical judgment requires knowledge of both nursing process and problem-specific facts (e.g., how health problems usually present and how they're usually managed).

▶ In the hospital setting, you might encounter few nursing diagnoses being formally addressed because hospitals usually focus only on problems that must be resolved in order for the person to be discharged from the hospital. In community and long-term care settings, you'll see more nursing diagnoses being addressed because there is more time, more family involvement, and nursing care focuses more on optimum wellness, than simply curing disease. Page 46 discusses the difference between nursing diagnoses and collaborative problems.

▶ Display 3–2 (page 49) provides the list of nursing diagnoses accepted for clinical testing by the North American Nursing Diagnosis Association (NANDA). Because the listed diagnoses are in various stages of development, and because some are controversial, I recommend that if you're a beginner, ask your instructor which diagnoses you should learn first.

▶ Nursing diagnoses are best identified by using a nursing model to collect and organize data. Tables 3–2 (page 47) and 3–3 (page 48) show two commonly used nursing models.

▶ Collaborative problems usually involve problems with structure or function of organs or systems. For this reason, they're best identified by using a body system approach to organizing data (see Fig. 3–2, page 52).

▶ Identifying both nursing diagnoses and collaborative problems is essential to developing a comprehensive nursing plan of care.

▶ Figure 3–3 (page 56) provides a decision-making model designed to help students decide whether an act is within their scope of practice.

▶ An essential nursing role in relation to collaborative problems is that of predicting, preventing, detecting, and managing *potential complications*. Display 3–3 (page 54) lists commonly encountered collaborative problems and their related potential complications.

▶ When you identify a collaborative problem, you must: (1) Make sure the physician is aware of the signs and symptoms. (2) Determine responses to medical treatment (is the patient responding as expected?). (3) Initiate collaborative and independent interventions as indicated by physician's orders and other applicable plans of care.

▶ Display 3–7 (page 62) offers a common system used to set immediate priorities. Consistently using the same method to set priorities helps you form habits that help you to be systematic and avoid missing key priorities.

▶ Decision-making in nursing is influenced by broad and specific standards. National standards for practice provide broad standards that address how nurses are generally expected to plan and deliver care. Facility and national guidelines are valuable tools to help you make care decisions.

▶ Standards and guidelines aren't meant to be followed *blindly*. An essential part of decision-making is using critical thinking to recognize when the situation at hand *differs* from the guide. You must carefully compare your patient's data with the information presented in the guideline, and decide whether the guidelines are indeed applicable to your specific patient.

▶ Developing clinical judgment takes time, and requires a commitment to study common health problems (nursing diagnoses and collaborative problems) and come prepared to the clinical setting. Pages 58–63 offer 10 strategies for developing effective clinical judgment.

▶ Display 3–5 (page 59) answers the eight key critical thinking questions presented in Chapter 2 in relation to clinical judgment.

OTHER PERSPECTIVES

Occasionally we hold a person's life in our hands; almost always his dignity.
   Leah Curtin.

OTHER PERSPECTIVES

.... the hospital is a dangerous place. It's the unusual patient who escapes without at least one scar: a phlebitis from an intravenous line, a miserable morning undergoing a poorly thought out barium enema, anxiety over the when and why of the next blood drawing, the emptiness of disenfranchisement from decisions affecting his own integrity and sanity. One must therefore be sure the hospitalized patient belongs in the hospital; as soon as the patient can function at home safely and comfortably, let him go.
   Fishman, M., et al. (1991). Medicine. Philadelphia: J.B. Lippincott.

End-of-Chapter Exercises

Instructions:

Limit responses to

2–5 sentences.

Example responses for these exercises can be found in the *Response Key,* which begins on page 136.

1. Figure 3–3 (page 56) provides a model to help students decide whether an act is within their scope of practice. Using this model, explain how you would decide if you could irrigate a nasogastric tube.

2. Consistently using the same method to set priorities helps you form *habits* that help you to be systematic and avoid missing key priorities. How can the mnemonics ABC'S and MAA-U-AR help you remember a system for setting priorities?

3. In the hospital setting, you might encounter fewer nursing diagnoses being addressed than in the community setting. Why?

4. An important aspect of developing clinical judgment is being willing to recognize the importance of caring (being willing to place great importance on the wants and needs of patients and their significant others). Keeping this in mind, what might you suspect has happened in the following dialogue between two nurses who are caring for a critically injured child?

   On-coming nurse: How is the family doing?

   Off-going nurse: They seem to be fine. They're sticking to visiting hours and have been in to visit 15 minutes this morning and 15 minutes this afternoon.

5. Complete the pre-chapter self-test, which has been reproduced below.

   a. Discuss how critical thinking in nursing is similar to and different from critical thinking in any situation.

   b. Define critical thinking in nursing and give four nursing situations when critical thinking is required.

   c. Name two major goals of nursing and discuss their implications for critical thinking.

   d. Explain how your level of knowledge and expertise (novice or expert) influences your ability to think critically.

   e. Discuss the relationship of the nursing process to critical thinking.

   f. Describe clinical judgment as addressed by Tanner (1983) and delBueno (1994).

   g. Identify a system for determining immediate priorities.

   h. Explain how national and facility standards are used as aids to decision-making.

   i. Describe five key strategies for developing clinical judgment.

Critical Thinking in Nursing:
Beyond Clinical Judgment

This chapter at a glance . . .

Why Read This Chapter?

PRE-CHAPTER SELF-TEST

Read the objectives listed below and decide whether you can readily achieve each one. If you can, skip this chapter, and go on to Chapter 5. Don't be concerned if you can't meet any of the objectives at this time. We'll come back to this self-test at the end of the chapter, so you'll get a second chance.

O B J E C T I V E S

1. Explain why nurses are frequently faced with moral and ethical issues.

2. Explain what is meant by the statement, "Moral and ethical issues sometimes have no right answers."

3. Make a prudent decision when deciding how to best help clients resolve moral and ethical issues.

4. Give three responsibilities of beginning nurses in relation to nursing research.

5. Use critical thinking to create a teaching plan.

6. Address the roles of memorizing and reasoning in teaching ourselves.

7. Name four things you must be knowledgeable about to increase your test scores, and explain why knowing this information is beneficial.

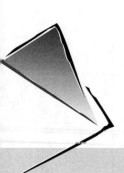

A B S T R A C T

This chapter continues the discussion of critical thinking in nursing from Chapter 3. It addresses the five remaining categories of critical thinking that are essential to nursing, but require different approaches (clinical reasoning, discussed in Chapter 3, was the first category addressed). The categories covered in this chapter are: moral and ethical reasoning, nursing research, teaching ourselves, teaching others, and test-taking.

Having defined critical thinking in nursing and examined how to develop clinical judgment, let's go on to examine the five other categories of critical thinking that are essential to nursing practice:

- Moral and ethical reasoning
- Nursing research
- Teaching others
- Teaching ourselves
- Test-taking

Let's begin with moral and ethical reasoning.

Moral and Ethical Reasoning

We know nurses are frequently faced with issues requiring moral and ethical reasoning. We're committed to giving humanistic care—we must try to allow people to make health care decisions based on their own values. However, sometimes this creates moral and ethical problems. For example, suppose you're caring for a woman who is an IV drug user and HIV-positive. As a nurse, you must provide compassionate, nonjudgmental care, right? But what if, during discussions about discharge, she insists that it's not her problem if other people choose to use her needles? Would it be correct to withhold judgment about this type of attitude? The answer is: *No.* It would be your moral and ethical responsibility to indicate that this type of behavior is unfair to others, and that the woman must not allow people to share her needles.

In the real world, the terms *moral reasoning* and *ethical reasoning* are used interchangeably. However, there is a slight difference between these two terms. Moral reasoning refers to judgments made based on personal standards of right and wrong (e.g., "I believe it's wrong to prolong life when death is inevitable"). Ethical reasoning usually refers to judgments made based on standards derived from the study of specific moral choices *made by people in relationships with others* (e.g., "While I personally believe prolonging life when death is inevitable is morally wrong, it's unethical for a nurse to influence client and family decisions about life and death, based on personal standards of right and wrong. Therefore, I won't voice my personal opinion about prolonging life").

Here's another example:

Case Scenario

■ Suppose you're admitting a young woman who is freely and knowledgeably seeking a tubal ligation. *Morally* (according to your personal standards), you feel sterilization is wrong. However, as a nurse, you realize that *ethically* this woman has a right to make this choice, and that it would be inappropriate for you to tell her sterilization is wrong, or for you to try to get her to change her mind.

So how *do* you make decisions about moral and ethical issues? The answer is: With great difficulty. Okay, so I'm only kidding—sometimes the issues are clear-cut, and it's not so difficult. But it's not unusual to be faced with situations in which there are no *right* answers. Rather, each answer has its own merits and weaknesses, and it's difficult to say that one is really better than another.

Moral and ethical problems may be divided into three categories (Jameton, 1984):

- **Moral uncertainty:** You aren't sure of which moral principles or values apply. *Example:* A patient asks you whether you think his doctor is a good doctor. You don't think the doctor is very competent. Do you tell him?
- **Moral dilemma:** You're faced with a situation in which you have two (or more) choices available, but none of them seem satisfactory. *Example:* A doctor tells *you* she's sure your friend has cancer, but tells *your friend,* "I won't know anything until the diagnosis is made by the lab, next week." When your friend begs you to tell him what the doctor knows, what do you do? If you tell him you don't know, you're lying. If you tell him what the doctor told you, you risk breaking his trust in his physician.
- **Moral distress:** You know the right thing to do, but institutional constraints make it nearly impossible to do what is right. *Example:* Mr. Potts is critically ill and you don't know if he'll survive. He's on a unit where there are strict rules against children visiting. He begs you to allow his children to come to his room's door so that he can wave to them. You believe seeing the children will make a significant difference in Mr. Potts' state of mind, and know a way you can sneak the children up without anyone knowing. What do you do?

To help you make these types of decisions, below are steps for making moral and ethical judgments.

Steps for Moral and Ethical Reasoning

1. **Clearly identify the issue based on the perspectives of the *key players* involved.** For example, Mrs. Pizzi, an elderly woman who lives alone, tells you she doesn't want her leg amputated, and that she'd rather die than live as an amputee. Her daughter tells you her mother is incompetent to make this decision. The problem is, who has the right to make this decision? Is Mrs. Pizzi competent? Does she have the right to refuse surgery? Does the daughter have the right to overrule her mother?

2. **Recognize your personal values and how they may influence your ability to participate in health care decision-making.** For example, in Mrs. Pizzi's case, do you believe no one has the right to refuse life-saving surgery? If so, how would this affect your ability to help Mrs. Pizzi with this decision? If you can't be objective, let your supervisor know so that another caregiver can assist with decision-making.

3. **Identify the alternatives.** For example, is it possible to delay this decision? Would Mrs. Pizzi be willing to have the surgery if the daughter commits to caring for her? Could social services help? Should we contact an expert in ethics?

4. **Determine the outcomes of the alternatives.** For example, if the decision is delayed, will it be detrimental to health? Would the daughter indeed be able to care for her mother?

5. **List the alternatives, and rate them according to which would produce least harm or greatest good, based on the *client's* values.** To do so, don't consider good versus bad. Instead, ask where each fits on the following scale:*

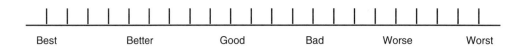

| Best | Better | Good | Bad | Worse | Worst |

The above scale will help you distinguish between choices, which, at first glance, might seem equally moral.

6. **Develop a plan of action that will facilitate the best choices.** In situations where the choices are all good, choose the one that is the

---

*From THE ART OF THINKING: A GUIDE TO CRITICAL AND CREATIVE THOUGHT, 3rd Edition by Vincent Ryan Ruggiero. Copyright © 1991 by HarperCollins Publishers, Inc. Reprinted by permission.

greater good. In situations where none of the choices are really good, choose the one that is the *lesser evil.*

7. **Put the plan into action, and monitor the response closely.**

To complete this section on moral and ethical reasoning, study Display 4–1, which answers key critical thinking questions in relation to moral and ethical decision-making.

Display 4–1 **Moral and Ethical Reasoning: Key Questions**

1. **What's the goal of my thinking?** To identify an ethically prudent course of action.
2. **What are the circumstances?** Circumstances vary: *Who's* involved? *What's* the issue and *what's* influencing its presentation (*when, where,* and *how* did the issue develop)? What are the morally significant variables present (e.g., beliefs, values, and preferences of the participants; cultural, religious, and economic considerations; interests of all involved parties)?
3. **What knowledge is required?** Required knowledge includes: familiarity with ethical theory and related principles, standards of care, professional codes of ethics (e.g., American Nurses Association Code of Ethics, *Patient's Bill of Rights,* listed in Appendix F, pages 163–166). You must also be familiar with a framework for ethical decision-making (see page 72), have good communication skills, and be clearly aware of the circumstances, as addressed in No. 2 above.
4. **How much room is there for error?** Room for error *varies* according to the consequences of the decision. For example, in which situation below do you think you have more room for error?
   a. You're deliberating about a patient's capacity to make an informed, voluntary decision about stopping life-sustaining therapies.
   b. You're deliberating about a patient's capacity to make an informed, voluntary decision about choosing among chemotherapies with different probabilities of success and side effects.
   If you thought *b,* you're correct. In situation *a,* you're deciding whether the person should live or die, leaving very little room for error. In situation *b,* as in many ethical problems, there may be no *right* answer. Rather, each answer has its own merits and risks with an equally uncertain outcome.
5. **How much time do I have?** Time frame for decision-making is also a factor of the consequences of the decision at hand. For example, if the parents of a sick child withhold consent for treatment, there's more time to deliberate if the child's life isn't in immediate jeopardy.
6. **What resources can help me?** Human resources include: clinical ethicists, ethics committees, clinical nurse educators, nursing faculty, facility policies on ethics, and librarians. Other resources include: Hastings Center,* *Hastings Report,* articles, ethics texts, computer data base, and professional ethics codes (e.g., American [or Canadian] Nurses Association Codes, American Medical Association Codes).

| Display 4–1 | Moral and Ethical Reasoning: Key Questions (*continued*) |

7. **Whose perspectives *must* be considered?** The most significant perspective to consider is that of the patient. Other important perspectives include: the family and significant others, caregivers, and relevant third parties (e.g., insurers); the perspectives of professional groups who have addressed the issues (e.g., those who have developed professional ethics codes as above, and the Hastings Center).

8. **What's influencing my thinking?** Thinking may be influenced by conscious or unconscious bias, discrimination, personal motives, or fear of legal liability (e.g., "I've got to restrain this person or he may fall, and I'll be sued"). Thinking may also be influenced by any of the factors listed in Table 2–1, Factors Influencing Critical Thinking (page 21).

*The Hastings Center, a nonprofit organization that carries out educational and research programs on ethics in medicine, life sciences, and professions, publishes the *Hastings Report* every 2 months. They can be contacted at 255 Elm Road, Briarcliff Manor, NY 10510.

Answers to questions provided by Carol Taylor, Ph.D. Candidate, MSN, Clinical Ethicist and Assistant Professor, Nursing, Georgetown University, Washington, DC.

Nursing Research

Based on strict rules of the scientific method, conducting research is one of the most rigorous and disciplined examples of critical thinking in nursing. Researchers must have a variety of critical thinking skills, from knowing how to clearly identify the problem or issue to be studied, to how to collect and analyze data. They must be able to consider *what* they see and the meaning *behind* what they see.

As in many professions, nursing research is accomplished by a comparatively small group of dedicated, highly qualified nurses who are willing to commit themselves to a lengthy, sometimes costly process.

So, you might wonder, "If research is conducted by a relatively small group of expert nurses, how important is it for beginning nurses?" The answer is: *Very important*. Research is essential to advancing nursing practice. It helps us generate a body of knowledge that provides a scientific basis for planning, predicting, and controlling the outcomes of nursing practice (Burns and Grove, 1993). Its importance is emphasized by the inclusion of *using research* as a standard of performance set forth by the American Nurses Association (ANA) (see Standard VII in Appendix E, page 162). By listing research as a *standard of performance*, the ANA sends the message that all nurses are expected to use research findings whenever appropriate.

Let's consider the questions, "What is the role of beginning nurses in relation to research?" and "How do you decide whether research findings can be safely used?"

Questions and Answers on Beginning Nurses' Research Role

1. **What is the role of beginning nurses in relation to nursing research?** Beginning nurses have four main responsibilities:
   a. **To think analytically about the situations they encounter and seek out research results that might improve nursing care.** For example, If you frequently care for people with postoperative leg edema after heart bypass surgery, you might think, "I wonder if there are any research studies explaining why this happens and what can be done about it?" To answer this question, you might simply be able to consult your instructor, a clinical nurse educator, or nurse researcher. Even if you don't have time to go to the library, often these people will help you.
   b. **To raise questions about their practice that might prompt a researcher to formulate a question to guide a study.** For example, you could ask your supervisor, "Since we seem to be having an increase in infections, would it be worthwhile to study whether our procedure for hand-washing is really effective?"
   c. **To help researchers collect data.** If you're asked to record certain information in the clinical area, it's your professional responsibility to do so, diligently and accurately, as long as it doesn't interfere with nursing care.
   d. **To continue to acquire and share knowledge related to research.** We must constantly be asking ourselves questions like, "Am I making time to become familiar with research related to the clinical situations in which I'm involved?" and "Do I interact with others (peers, educators) to learn more about research?" For those of you who find reading research articles tedious, get started by talking with peers and educators, or perhaps joining a journal club. This helps you to learn in a dynamic, stimulating environment. Once you learn the basics, meeting your responsibilities in relation to research becomes easier, more interesting, and even an enjoyable challenge!

2. **If I have limited knowledge of research, how do I know whether there are research studies I should be using in my practice?** The following will help you answer this question.
   a. **Recognize research findings must not be used indiscriminately.** Before you can use research results, you must decide whether the study is valid and reliable (whether it was conducted in such a way that you can trust that the results are accurate). For example, how often have you heard a commercial that proclaims, "In a recent research study, our product was proven to be more effective than the other leading products." Do you believe every one of these commercials? Probably not. As independent thinkers, you must always ask questions to determine whether you can apply the results of *any* research study.
   b. **Search the literature for research articles related to your**

area of practice. The first time you do this, take a partner with you to the library, and tackle the search collaboratively.

c. **Choose titles that sound as though they'd help you manage the problems you frequently encounter better** (e.g., research on pain management).

d. **Scan first to eliminate irrelevant articles, then read the ones that seem as though they'd be most useful.** Learning how to scan then read research articles efficiently helps you avoid becoming overwhelmed with trying to do too much at one time. To learn how to choose relevant research articles more easily, and how to decide whether you know enough to use a specific study's results, review Displays 4–2 and 4–3.

Quality Improvement

It would be a mistake to discuss nursing research without taking at least a few moments to specifically address quality improvement (QI). QI is perhaps the most frequent type of research encountered in the clinical setting. Almost every facility has a department whose responsibility it is to conduct studies to improve care quality. By continually monitoring how care is given and what results are achieved, researchers in quality improvement make a "grass roots" impact on nursing care—they gather and analyze data within their facility, and often change policies based on their studies' results. For example, more than a few facilities, through ongoing quality improvement studies, have documented that delays in medications coming from pharmacy cause a significant increase in length of hospital

Display 4–2	How to Scan, Then Read Research Articles

Scanning to find useful research articles saves time by helping you eliminate irrelevant articles without having to read them in their entirety.

1. **Read the abstract first: This summarizes the issues, methods, and results.** If the abstract isn't applicable to your clinical problem, you might choose to read no further.

2. **If the abstract sounds applicable, skip to the end of the article,** then scan the article by reading the information under the following headings, in the order listed below:
   a. Summary (may also be listed as "Conclusions")
   b. Discussion
   c. Nursing Implications
   d. Suggestions For Further Research
   You may able to eliminate articles just by reading any of the above headings.

3. **If the information you've scanned is relevant, go on to read the entire study.** Give yourself plenty of time, and don't be discouraged if you find sections you don't understand. Instead, take notes on what you *do* understand. Come back to the more difficult sections at another time, after getting help from an expert or textbook (or both).

Display 4-3	Questions to Ask Yourself to Decide Whether You Know Enough About a Research Article to Use the Results

1. **Do I understand:**
   - What's already known about the topic (this is usually found under the heading of "Literature Review")?
   - What the researchers studied, why they studied it, and how they studied it?
   - What they found out?
   - What the results mean, and how they might be used in my particular clinical situation?
2. **Do I know how the results of this study compare with the results of other, similar studies?** If other studies produced similar findings, the probability that the results are *reliable* increases.
3. **What experts, references, or texts can help me analyze the details of this study and decide whether the methods and results are reliable?** Before you use research findings, discuss the results with your supervisor.

stays. These documented results have caused facilities to change or create policies to make sure medications come to the units in a timely fashion.

Your responsibilities in relation to QI are the same as the previously listed responsibilities for research.

To complete this section, review Display 4–4, which answers key critical thinking questions in relation to nursing research.

Teaching Others

Creative critical thinking is essential to teach people the information they need to be independent. People today are discharged sicker and quicker than they were in the past, and many receive health care on an outpatient basis. Our teaching must be timely and effective. We must be able to clearly identify what *must* be learned, and then initiate a plan that draws on client strengths.

The following steps are provided to help you think critically about how to teach others:

1. **Get to know who you're teaching.**
   a. Assess people's readiness to learn: Ask what their biggest concerns are, and *listen.*
   b. Determine their preferred learning styles (e.g., doing, observing, listening, or reading). Encourage them to use their own best style. For example, if they're doers, have them start by *doing* something, like handling a syringe, if you're teaching injection technique. If they'd rather read, start by giving them a pamphlet.
2. **Encourage them to ask questions, get involved, and let you know how they'd like to learn.** For example, you could say, "Let me know if you have a better way of learning this...not everyone learns the same way."

Display 4–4	**Nursing Research: Key Questions**

1. **What's the goal of my thinking?** To learn more about an issue or problem of concern to nursing by conducting a study that's as scientifically sound and reliable as possible (it might be difficult to study some issues or problems *scientifically*).

2. **What are the circumstances?** Circumstances vary: What's the issue or problem to be studied? What are the ethical concerns? Considering all factors (e.g., availability of research subjects, budgetary concerns, practicality), what's the best method to conduct the study?

3. **What knowledge is required?** Required knowledge includes: familiarity with the topic, previous research on the topic, research methods, and (for some research designs) statistical analysis. You also need to be familiar with the following library resources: indexes, catalogs, computer search services, inter-library loan services, circulation department, reference department, and audiovisual services.

4. **How much room is there for error?** Every effort is made to minimize possibility of error, or the results are invalid. However, the room for error *varies* depending on how the research results might be used. For example, in which situation below do you think you have more room for error?
   a. You're conducting a study to determine what colors have a calming effect so that hospitals can choose calming colors for their walls.
   b. You're conducting a study to determine the best ways to prevent postoperative breathing complications so that you can include these methods in facility guidelines for postoperative care.

   If you thought a, you're correct. Little harm can occur if you're incorrect about the best colors, but if you're incorrect about how to best manage postoperative breathing complications, lives may be in jeopardy.

5. **How much time do I have?** The time frame depends on the research design (may be as short as a few days to as long as decades). Some nurses must complete their research as a requirement for a course, which limits their time to the length of the course.

6. **What resources can help me?** Human resources include: nurse researchers, clinical nurse educators, clinical nurse specialists, faculty, preceptors, peers, journal clubs, librarians. Other resources include: research texts, journal articles, computer data bases.

7. **Whose perspectives *must* be considered?** The most significant perspective to consider is that of the *subjects* involved in the research (patients, families, etc.), with great consideration given to rights of privacy and efficient health care. Other perspectives are those of the data collectors, the researchers, and interested third parties (e.g., parties funding the study).

8. **What's influencing my thinking?** Thinking may be influenced by vested interest in results. It may also be influenced by any of the factors listed in Table 2–1, Factors Influencing Critical Thinking (page 21).

3. **Reduce anxiety by offering support.** An example is saying something like, "Everyone is nervous when first learning to change dressings, but once you've done it a couple of times, it will be much easier."

4. **Minimize distractions, and teach at appropriate times.** For example, pick a quiet room, and choose times when the learners are likely to be comfortable and rested.

5. **Use pictures, diagrams, and illustrations.** These visual aids enhance comprehension and are better remembered.

6. **Use analogies and metaphors to create a "mental visual."** One example is, "Insulin is like a key that opens the cell's door to allow sugar to enter. If you don't have a key (insulin), the sugar can't get into the cell. The cell starves, and sugar accumulates in the blood."

7. **Encourage people to paraphrase using their own words— words that help them remember.** For example, someone might say, "I need to have three things: The *soaking-dressing stuff*, the *scrubbing stuff*, and the *after-dressing stuff*."

8. **For complex information, consider using the explain-it-to-me-as-if-I-were-a-four-year-old approach (keep it simple).***

9. **Tune into your learners' responses, and change the pace, techniques, or content if needed.** For example, if they've forgotten important content, take time to review it; if they don't seem to understand what you're saying, write it down or draw a picture.

10. **Summarize key points and don't leave learners empty handed.** Even the best learners may have trouble remembering what they've just been taught. Give them the important points in writing so they can refresh their memory later.

To complete this section, review Display 4–5 (next page), which answers key critical thinking questions in relation to teaching others.

Teaching Ourselves

As addressed in Chapter 1, the challenges of nursing today require us to know how to teach ourselves. To be successful, we must take a proactive approach to learning. We need to be able to identify what it is we must learn, and then find ways to learn it efficiently.

Using critical thinking when we learn, or reasoning our way through the learning process, helps us connect with our own unique way of making information *ours*. Richard Paul, author of *Critical Thinking: How to Prepare Students for a Rapidly Changing World,* describes using reasoning to learn as going something like this:

---

* The explain-it-to-me-as-if-I-were-a-four-year-old approach comes from the movie *Philadelphia,* in which the lawyer tries to understand all his clients' situations by telling them, "Explain it to me as if I were a four year old."

Display 4–5	Teaching Others: Key Questions

1. **What's the goal of my thinking?** To help others gain required information efficiently.
2. **What are the circumstances?** Circumstances vary: *Who's* involved (e.g., adult; child; person with limited learning skills, language barriers)? *What* must be learned? Is it simple or complex? Does it simply require knowledge, or are there motor skills to be mastered?
3. **What knowledge is required?** Required knowledge includes: familiarity with content to be taught, communication skills, teaching and learning principles. You must also be clearly aware of the circumstances, as addressed in No. 2 above.
4. **How much room is there for error?** Room for error *varies* according to consequences of what happens if the learner doesn't master the information. For example, in which situation below do you think you have more room for error?
   a. You're teaching insulin injection technique to someone who's basically healthy and whose daughter is an ICU nurse who's willing to monitor injection technique at home.
   b. You're teaching insulin injection technique to someone who has a compromised immune system and lives alone with no relatives.
   If you thought *a*, you're correct. If the person in situation *b* goes home without mastering insulin technique, he may not manage his diabetes, and he may develop an infection. Therefore, you must be *sure* his injection technique is meticulous.
5. **How much time do I have?** The time frame for teaching depends on outcome setting (goal setting) during planning. For example, if by day 3, the person is expected to be discharged, you have 3 days to teach the required information or home care visits may be required.
6. **What resources can help me?** Human resources include: clinical nurse educators, clinical nurse specialists, preceptors, more experienced nurses, peers, librarians, and other health care professionals (pharmacists, nutritionists, physical therapists, physicians). The learners are also valuable resources (it's not unusual for them to be the ones who can best identify what must be learned and how they can best learn it). Other resources include: texts, articles, computerized learning packages, pamphlets, audio visuals, facility documents (e.g., teaching guidelines, standards of care).
7. **Whose perspectives *must* be considered?** The most significant perspective to consider is that of the learners: How ready are they to learn? What is it they think they need to learn? How do they learn best? What are motivating factors for them to learn (e.g., some people need a deadline or a test)? Another perspective to consider is your own (e.g., how do *you* feel you can best teach the material?).
8. **What's influencing my thinking?** A major influencing factor is whether the learners think they can learn, and whether *you* think you can be successful in helping them (both can be self-fulfilling prophecies). Thinking may also be influenced by any of the factors listed in Table 2–1, Factors Influencing Critical Thinking (page 21).

Let's see, how can I understand this? Is it to be understood on the model of this experience or that? Shall I think of it in this way or that? Let me see. Ah, I think I see. It's just so . . . but, no, not exactly. Let me try again. Perhaps I can understand it from this point of view, by interpreting it thus. OK, now I think I'm getting it. . . . (Paul, 1993, p. 305.)

When you encounter new information, take charge and reason your way through the learning experience. Make your goal to have critical thinking pervade your learning practices. Be confident in your ability to learn. Question deeply, and use your preferred learning style. Remember, you are your own best teacher.

Memorizing Effectively

As much as experts emphasize that critical thinking is *more* than memorizing (remembering facts), learning how to memorize effectively enhances your ability to think critically: You must be able to recall facts to progress to higher levels of thinking, such as knowing how to apply and analyze information. For example, if you aren't able to *recall* what *normal* health assessment findings are, you won't be able to *analyze* your patient's data to decide whether there are any *abnormal* findings.

Some disciplines require more memorization than others, Nursing is a discipline that requires a considerable amount of memorization, especially in the beginning. The following strategies are suggested to help you memorize effectively:

1. **Try to understand before you try to memorize.** Once you make sense of the information, you'll begin to realize what's most important, and how it can best be organized to help you remember it.
2. **Don't try to memorize everything.** Take the time to identify what's most important, then separate this information from all the other information. This prevents you from trying to memorize too much. Your brain can only take so much new information at a time.
3. **Work to find relationships between the facts**, **rather than trying to just remember a list of facts.** Groups of information are more readily remembered than isolated facts. The process of trying to understand how the facts relate to each other will also help you *remember* the facts.
4. **Create a memory hook.** Put the information into context. For example, if you've looked after someone with the diagnosis you're studying, visualize the patient and how the situation compared with the information you're studying (the patient then becomes your memory hook). If you don't have a real situation to connect with, play around with the information until something comes to mind that helps you remember (a rhyme, a picture, a story, a mnemonic). For example, consider the following techniques:

a. **Use a mnemonic** (organize what you're trying to remember in such a way that each word's first letter makes a real or nonsensical word). For example, look at the two following mnemonics:

TACT helps you remember what you should be monitoring when giving medications:

T = Therapeutic effect
A = Adverse reactions
C = Contraindications
T = Toxicity/overdose

PERRL (*P*upils *E*qually *R*ound, and *R*eactive to *L*ight) helps you remember that you check the pupils to make sure they react equally to light when doing a neurologic assessment.

b. **Use an acrostic** (create a catchy phrase that helps you remember the first letters of the information you're trying to remember). For example:

*M*aggie *C*hewed *N*uts *E*very *P*lace *S*he *W*ent provides the first letter of things you need to assess when performing a neurovascular assessment:

*M*ovement, *C*olor, *N*umbness, *E*dema, *P*ulses, *S*ensation, *W*armth.

5. **In addition to using your preferred learning style, use as many senses as possible.** If you use other senses together with your preferred style, you'll remember even more. For example, use visual and auditory senses together by reading aloud, or use all three senses by saying the words as you write and read them.

6. **Put the information on tape.** Tapes can be played almost anywhere, anytime. Those minutes driving, walking, or riding a bicycle can be valuable time to load information into long-term memory.

7. **Organize the information, then see if you can organize it a *different* way.** By mentally using the information in different ways, you'll remember it better.

8. **Review the information briefly before going to sleep.** Studies show that even if you're a "morning person," information moves into long-term memory better if reviewed late in the day, immediately before going to bed.

9. **Use the information and quiz yourself periodically ("use it or lose it").** Remember, just because you can recognize information in your notes, it doesn't mean you'll be able to *recall* the information *without* your notes.

10. **Know yourself and use self-discipline.** Identify the circumstances that help you retain information, and plan your schedule to include those circumstances. For example, if you study better in the morning, be sure you go to bed early enough so that you can get up early and feel rested; if you're easily distracted or side-tracked, plan to go to the library, or put a "Don't Disturb" sign on your door.

For a list of helpful references for learning how to teach yourself efficiently, see Display 4–6.

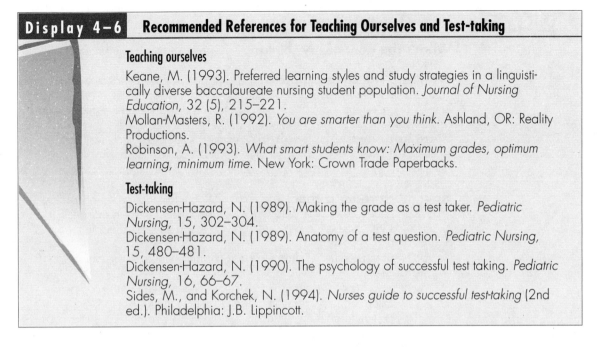

Display 4–6   **Recommended References for Teaching Ourselves and Test-taking**

Teaching ourselves

Keane, M. (1993). Preferred learning styles and study strategies in a linguistically diverse baccalaureate nursing student population. *Journal of Nursing Education*, 32 (5), 215–221.

Mollan-Masters, R. (1992). *You are smarter than you think*. Ashland, OR: Reality Productions.

Robinson, A. (1993). *What smart students know: Maximum grades, optimum learning, minimum time*. New York: Crown Trade Paperbacks.

Test-taking

Dickensen-Hazard, N. (1989). Making the grade as a test taker. *Pediatric Nursing*, 15, 302–304.

Dickensen-Hazard, N. (1989). Anatomy of a test question. *Pediatric Nursing*, 15, 480–481.

Dickensen-Hazard, N. (1990). The psychology of successful test taking. *Pediatric Nursing*, 16, 66–67.

Sides, M., and Korchek, N. (1994). *Nurses guide to successful test-taking* (2nd ed.). Philadelphia: J.B. Lippincott.

To complete this section, review Display 4–7 (next page), which answers key critical thinking questions in relation to teaching ourselves.

Test-taking

The final critical thinking category we'll cover is test-taking. Test-taking doesn't stop after school or state board exams. As we progress through our careers, most of us face at least one test a year (e.g., almost all of us take the annual cardiopulmonary resuscitation recertification test).

Test-taking can be truly anxiety producing, and often frustrating. We've all been in the position of knowing information well and not being able to perform on the test. Lots of us can reason *well* in real situations, but are stumped when it comes to reasoning our way to determine a correct *test* answer. Someone once said to me, "I need a real person and real situation to think well." If you're one of those people (as I am), this section should be helpful to you.

Using critical thinking to identify the best way to prepare for and take tests can reduce your anxiety and improve your test scores. Being successful at test-taking requires more than knowledge about the *content*. It also requires you to know yourself, know about the test format, and know test-taking *skills*. The following strategies are suggested to help you improve your test scores:

1. **Know yourself.** Identify your usual test-taking behaviors: For example, do you get overly anxious, do you frequently run out of time,

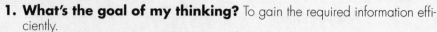

| Display 4–7 | **Teaching Ourselves: Key Questions** |

1. **What's the goal of my thinking?** To gain the required information efficiently.
2. **What are the circumstances?** Circumstances vary: *What* must you learn? Does it simply require knowledge, or are there motor skills to master as well? Why must you learn it? How motivated are you to learn the information or tasks? What's your preferred learning style?
3. **What knowledge is required?** Required knowledge includes: knowledge of self (e.g., preferred learning styles, motivations), learning skills, critical thinking skills. You must also be clearly aware of the circumstances, as addressed in No. 2 above.
4. **How much room is there for error?** Room for error *varies* according to the consequences of what happens if you don't learn the information. For example, in which situation below do you think you have more room for error?
   a. You need to prepare for an open book exam on nursing care of respiratory problems.
   b. You need to master respiratory assessment and tracheal suctioning before you take care of someone with a tracheostomy tomorrow.
   If you said *a*, you're correct. The risk of harm to your patient leaves little room for error.
5. **How much time do I have?** The time frame for learning depends on when you'll need to use the information. But remember, your brain can only learn so much in one sitting.
6. **What resources can help me?** Human resources include: professionals specializing in how to learn, clinical nurse educators, preceptors, clinical nurse specialists, peers, and librarians. Other resources include: texts on content, texts on how to learn (see Display 4–6), articles, computerized learning packages, pamphlets, audio visuals.
7. **Whose perspectives *must* be considered?** The most significant perspective to consider is your *own*. How ready are you to learn? What is it you think you need to learn most? How do you learn best? What usually motivates you to learn? Other perspectives to consider are those of your teachers (e.g., they may be better at teaching one way or another).
8. **What's influencing my thinking?** A major influencing factor is whether you think you can master the information (this can be a self-fulfilling prophecy). Thinking may also be influenced by any of the factors listed in Table 2–1, Factors Influencing Critical Thinking (page 21).

OTHER PERSPECTIVES

Heightened awareness often precedes a change in behavior. For example, once you know you tend to make assumptions, you soon begin to double-check your thinking.

Carol Matz.

are you more successful at one type of test than another? Seek help for areas you'd like to change (see Display 4–6 on page 83 for helpful references).

2. **Know the test plan.** Find out what types of questions (multiple choice, short-answer, essay) are going to be used, and what information is most important to study. If the faculty doesn't share this information, review course objectives and text objectives and summaries—often these will help you decide.

3. **Start preparing with an attitude of "I can do this—I just have to figure out how."** You are capable. Sometimes you need to remind yourself of this to acquire the positive attitude we all know is so important.

4. **Get organized and plan ahead.** Decide what you need to study, what your resources are (notes, books, tutors), and when and how you'll prepare for the test.

5. **Learn how to read questions**: How to identify the background statement, the stem, and the key words (see Display 4–8). This helps

---

Display 4–8	**Components of a Test Question**

1. **The background statement(s).** The statements or phrases that facilitate answering the question (e.g., the words *not* in bold in the example test question below):

    You're caring for someone who has severe asthma, is wheezing loudly, is confused, and can't sleep. You check the orders, and note that a sedative can be given for sleeplessness. **Knowing the possible effects of giving a sedative to an asthmatic, what would you do?**
    a. Give the sedative to help the patient relax.
    b. Withhold the sedative because it aggravates asthma.
    c. Withhold the sedative because it may cause excessive somnolence.
    d. Give the sedative, but monitor the patient carefully.

2. **The stem.** A phrase that asks or states the intent of the question. For example, the words in bold in the example test question above.

3. **Key concepts.** The most important *concepts* addressed in the background statement(s) that help you answer the question. In the above example, the key concepts are: severe asthma, wheezing loudly, effects of giving a sedative to an asthmatic.

4. **Key word(s).** The words that *specify* what's being asked and what's happening. In the example above, the key words are: severe; loudly; confused. These words specify that the asthma problem is severe. "Would you do" specifies that you're being asked for an appropriate action to take.

5. **The options (choices).** These include one correct answer (called the *keyed response*) and three to five *distractors* (incorrect answers). In the example above, c is the keyed response, and the rest are distractors.

you choose the best response when given similar responses, and helps you make an educated guess when you're unsure whether any of the responses are appropriate.

6. **Practice, practice, practice,** answering the types of questions you expect to take on the test (e.g., practice multiple choice questions for state board exams). One of the reasons some of us don't do well on tests is because we don't take them every day. Often, answering discussion questions and end-of-chapter exercises are also good ways to practice. If you're going to take the test on a computer, practice on the computer. For state board exams, take a review course.

7. **Arrive early for warm-up.** Give yourself time to calm down, get focused, and mentally go through information you've decided is important. Reviewing practice questions is also a good way to get your brain in "test-taking" gear.

8. **If possible, skim the whole test and plan your approach.*** For example, you might begin by answering the types of questions you like before tackling types you don't like (e.g., you may like matching better than essay). Completing what you like and know first reduces anxiety and gets your brain in the "test-taking" mode before tackling more difficult questions.

9. **Focus on what you know.**
   a. Skip more difficult questions and come back to them later.* For example, put a question mark next to questions you *might* be able to answer, and an "X" next to the toughest questions. Go back to the "question mark questions" before the "X questions."
   b. For essay, jot down key points you know you want to address before writing your essay. When you're finished, check your essay to be sure you've hit all the major points and that you've been clear.
   c. For essay and short-answer questions, if you have time at the end, come back to these questions and ask yourself. "What else can I say?" or "What did I miss?"

10. **Let your instructor know if you don't understand a question.** You may not be allowed to ask questions during the test, but consider writing something like, "I wasn't sure if you meant. . . ." or ". . . so I'm answering the question assuming you meant. . . ." If allowed, write this on your answer sheet or flip the answer sheet over.

11. **When in doubt, don't change answers.** Studies show your first response is more likely to be correct.

12. **For case history questions:** Read questions about the case history first, then read the histories with the intent of looking for the answers.

---

*Some computer tests, like state board exams, don't allow for skimming, moving around in the test, or changing answers.

13. **When you're struggling to answer:** Consider whether sketching a picture or diagram will help you conceptualize the answer.

14. **Watch your time and note how the questions are weighted.** For example, if a question is worth 50% of your grade, you might want to save 50% of your time to work on that question.

15. **If you do poorly, don't think it's the end of the world.** Even the brightest, most knowledgeable minds have been known to fail tests (Einstein flunked algebra; Edison was considered unteachable). Instead, *do* something (e.g., explain your difficulty to your instructor; ask if there's some way you can prepare better, or if you can do extra credit work; determine resources that can help you; practice, practice, practice).

To complete this section, review Display 4–9 (next page), which answers key critical thinking questions in relation to test-taking.

Summary

This chapter examines five commonly encountered categories of critical thinking in nursing: moral and ethical reasoning, nursing research, teaching others, teaching ourselves, and test-taking. To solidify your knowledge of this chapter, read the following key points, and go on to complete the end-of-chapter exercises.

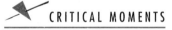

CRITICAL MOMENTS

Once I asked a nurse* if he wished he could do his charting by just dictating to a tape recorder. He responded, "Not really. When I write, I think." Then I asked, "What if you could dictate, then print out your notes and read them?" He responded, "Maybe then I'd like it because I could still evaluate my thoughts and see what I missed."
When charting, evaluate your thinking—look for flaws and correct them. When thinking about something important, put your thoughts down on paper. It helps you stay focused and *evaluate* thoughts as you write.

   *Julio Suarez, a staff nurse on the Bone Marrow Transplant Unit at Hahnemann Hospital in Philadelphia, PA.

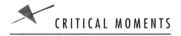

CRITICAL MOMENTS

Seek out mentors and role models—teachers, other nurses, friends, peers. They help you clarify your thoughts and set goals better than any textbook.

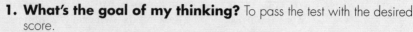

| Display 4-9 | Test-taking: Key Questions |

1. **What's the goal of my thinking?** To pass the test with the desired score.
2. **What are the circumstances?** Circumstances vary: How important is it for you to get your desired score? What content will be tested? What type of test is it (e.g., objective, subjective, open book, computerized)? On what type of tests do you perform best?
3. **What knowledge is required?** Required knowledge includes: knowledge of self (e.g., study habits, learning style, test-taking patterns). You must also be clearly aware of the circumstances, as addressed in No. 2 above.
4. **How much room is there for error?** Room for error *varies* according to the type of test to be taken and the consequences of what happens if you don't pass the test. For example, in which situation below do you think you have more room for error?
   a. You're going to take a mid-term exam in a course where you have a C minus average.
   b. You're going to take a weekly quiz in a course where at the mid-term you had an A average.
   Of course, *b* is the right answer.
5. **How much time do I have?** Time frame varies, as we all know!
6. **What resources can help me?** Human resources include: professionals specializing in learning and test-taking, peers. Other resources include: texts and articles on test-taking, review books (see Display 4-6).
7. **Whose perspectives *must* be considered?** Both your own perspective and that of whomever constructed the test must be considered. It's important to realize that the person who is testing you *wants* you to do well, but needs to feel comfortable that you've mastered the required content.
8. **What's influencing my thinking?** A major influencing factor is whether you think you can pass the test (this can be a self-fulfilling prophecy). Thinking may also be influenced by any of the factors listed in Table 2-1, Factors Influencing Critical Thinking (page 21).

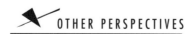

OTHER PERSPECTIVES

The significant problems we face today cannot be solved at the same level of thinking we were at when we created them.

Albert Einstein.

KEY POINTS

▶ This chapter continues the discussion of critical thinking in nursing from Chapter 3, addressing the five remaining categories of critical thinking (moral and ethical reasoning, nursing research, teaching ourselves, teaching others, and test-taking).

▶ The terms *moral reasoning* and *ethical reasoning* are often used interchangeably.

▶ It's not unusual to be faced with moral and ethical issues that have no *right* answer: Rather, each answer has its own merits and risks with an equally uncertain outcome.

▶ Moral and ethical problems may be divided into three categories: Moral uncertainty, moral dilemma, moral distress. These are discussed on page 71.

▶ To help you make these types of decisions, pages 72–73 present steps for making moral and ethical judgments.

▶ Display 4–1 (pages 73 and 74) answers key critical thinking questions in relation to moral and ethical reasoning.

▶ Based on strict rules of the scientific method, conducting nursing research is one of the most rigorous and disciplined examples of critical thinking in nursing.

▶ The ANA emphasizes the importance of using research by including using research in their standards of performance (Standard VII in Appendix E, page 162).

▶ Pages 75–76 provide questions and answers on beginning nurses' research roles and responsibilities. Display 4–2 (page 76) provides guidelines for scanning research articles efficiently.

▶ Research results must not be used indiscriminately. Display 4–3 (page 77) provides questions to ask to decide whether you know enough about the research study to use the results.

▶ Quality improvement (QI) is perhaps the most frequent type of research encountered in the clinical setting. QI studies involve continually monitoring how care is given and what results are achieved. Based on QI study results, hospitals often change or create policies to improve care quality.

▶ Display 4–4 (page 78) answers key critical thinking questions in relation to nursing research.

▶ Creative critical thinking is essential to finding ways to teach people the information they need to be independent. Our teaching must be timely and effective.

▶ Pages 77–79 provide steps to help you think critically about teaching others. Display 4–5 (page 80) answers key critical thinking questions in relation to teaching others.

▶ To be successful in nursing today, we must take a proactive approach to learning. We need to be able to identify what it is we must learn, and then find ways to learn it efficiently.

▶ Using critical thinking when we learn, or reasoning our way through the learning process, helps us connect with our own unique way of making information ours.

▶ Nursing is a discipline that requires a considerable amount of memorization. Pages 81–82 provide strategies for memorizing effectively.

▶ Display 4–7 (page 84) answers key critical thinking questions in relation to teaching ourselves.

▶ Test-taking doesn't stop after school or state board exams. As we progress through our careers, most of us face at least one test a year.

▶ Using critical thinking to identify the best way to prepare for and take tests can reduce your anxiety and improve your test scores.

▶ Being successful at test-taking requires more than knowledge about the content. It also requires you to know yourself (to identify ways of taking advantage of strengths and compensating for weaknesses), know about the test format (to identify ways of preparing for the test), and know test-taking skills (to make the most of what you know, and to make educated guesses when you're unsure).

▶ Pages 83–87 provide strategies for test-taking.

CRITICAL MOMENTS

When you want to know something well, offer to teach it to someone else. You learn and recall best what you teach someone else.

OTHER PERSPECTIVES

Nursing requires that nurses think critically while they're doing nursing. Thinking critically involves paying attention to how one is thinking as nursing care is accomplished. Nurses should ask themselves questions like, "What are my assumptions in this situation?" "Are they accurate?" "What additional information do I need?" "How can I look at this situation in a different way?" This kind of critical thinking can occur while doing, or it can occur after doing. The important part is that nurses observe how thinking occurs and how effective it is. Critical thinking following doing is often called reflective thinking. Thinking while doing is often called "thinking in action."

Joan Jenks.

End-of-Chapter Exercises

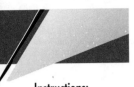

Instructions:

Limit responses to

2–5 sentences.

Example responses for these exercises can be found in the Response Key, which begins on page 136.

1. Explain why knowing how to teach others efficiently is essential to meeting the goals of nursing.
2. Explain what is meant by moral uncertainty, moral dilemmas, and moral distress.
3. Describe five strategies that can help you memorize more effectively.
4. Describe five strategies that can help you improve your test scores.
5. Complete the pre-chapter self-test, which has been reproduced below.
   a. Explain why nurses are frequently faced with moral and ethical issues.
   b. Explain what is meant by the statement, "Moral and ethical issues sometimes have no right answers."
   c. Make a prudent decision when deciding how to best help clients resolve moral and ethical issues. To complete this objective, consider the following situation: The Blanco's have cared for their 40-year-old daughter, Marilou, at home for 20 years, since she became totally comatose after a car accident. According to her physicians, all diagnostic studies performed indicate that Marilou has no brain functioning. The Blanco's are considering stopping tube feedings, and allowing her to die. Consider all the questions in Display 4–1 (pages 73 and 74), and decide how can you best help the Blanco's make this decision. (No response provided for this exercise in the Response Key.)
   d. Give three responsibilities of beginning nurses in relation to nursing research.
   e. Use critical thinking to create a teaching plan. To complete this objective, ask a fellow student something he or she would like to learn, and develop a teaching plan, using the teaching strategies provided on pages 77–79 (no response provided for this exercise in the Response Key).
   f. Address the roles of memorizing and reasoning in teaching ourselves.
   g. Name four things you must be knowledgeable about to increase your test scores, and explain why knowing this information is beneficial.

5

Practicing Critical Thinking Skills*

This chapter at a glance . . . .

---

* The wording of some of the names and definitions of the skills in this section varies slightly from that listed in Chapter 3 (page 31). This is because some of the skills are addressed in more detail in this section, and some of the skills are combined to facilitate learning how to use the skills within the framework of the nursing process.

Why Read This Chapter?

PRE-CHAPTER SELF-TEST

Read the objectives listed below and decide whether you can readily achieve each one. If you can, skip this chapter. If you can achieve only some of the objectives, complete only the sections you need to practice.

O B J E C T I V E S

1. Explain why each skill in this section promotes critical thinking (see skills listed on facing page).

2. Explain how each skill in this section is accomplished.

3. Identify five critical thinking skills you'd like to improve.

ABSTRACT

This chapter provides opportunities to practice critical thinking skills in nursing situations. It covers 16 skills that enhance critical thinking. Each skill is presented in the following format: name of the skill, definition of the skill, why the skill promotes critical thinking, how to accomplish the skill, and practice exercises.

Each skill in this section is presented as a *separate skill*. However, in actuality, these skills usually aren't used separately, or necessarily at any one particular step of the nursing process. Rather, in the real world, these skills are *inter-related,* often overlap, and are used at any stage of the nursing process. For example, as you're implementing a plan of care, you might *recognize inconsistencies* (Skill VIII) in the patient's response, and think to yourself, "Maybe we've made an *assumption*" (Skill I).

To keep the length of this section manageable, the focus is on applying critical thinking to *problem identification*. Although the focus is on problem identification, I don't intend to minimize the importance of looking for patient *strengths* and seeking ways to improve areas that are satisfactory but could be improved. Identifying patient strengths is essential to developing an efficient plan of care. Identifying ways to improve is essential for progress.

General Instructions

To get the most out of these exercises, don't try to do too many at one time. Some of these exercises, as in real life, are quite time consuming. The purpose of the exercises *isn't* to do them as quickly as possible. Rather, take your time, and get in touch with your thinking as you do them. If possible, get at least one other person to complete the exercises with you. You'll learn more by discussing the skills with others. The point of this section is not to provide one *right response*. Rather, it is to demonstrate critical thinking by providing several plausible responses, then choosing the one you think is best.

Some of these practice sections will require you to look up information in another textbook. This is especially true if your mental storehouse of problem-specific facts is limited: Critical thinking in nursing requires *application* of problem-specific facts (see Display 3–6 on page 61). If you encounter a disease or drug that you don't know, look it up before attempting to read on.

Before you start this section, be sure you've mastered the vocabulary below. These terms are listed in order of how they can best be learned, rather than alphabetically (you need to know the first term to understand the second term, and so on).

Required Vocabulary for Completing This Chapter

Nursing Diagnosis. See discussion beginning on page 45.

Collaborative Problem. See discussion beginning on page 45.

Definitive Diagnosis. The most specific, most correct diagnosis. For example, someone may be admitted with the diagnosis of respiratory distress. Then, after studies are completed, it may be decided that the definitive diagnosis is pneumonia. When the *most specific diagnosis* is identified, it makes it easier to identify specific interventions (actions) to treat the problem: This is true for both medical diagnoses and nursing diagnoses.

Risk Factor. Something known to contribute to, or be associated with, a specific problem (e.g., obesity is known to be a risk factor for hypertension).

Related Factor. See Risk Factor.

Potential Problem or Risk Diagnosis.[*] A problem or diagnosis that may occur because of certain risk factors present (e.g., someone who's on prolonged bed rest has a potential or risk for skin breakdown). Often used interchangeably with *high risk problem or diagnosis* (see below).

High Risk Problem or Diagnosis. A problem or diagnosis for which someone is *more* at risk than *others in the same situation.* For example, anyone on prolonged bed rest has a potential or risk for *Impaired Skin Integrity.* However, an elderly diabetic is *more* at risk for *Impaired Skin Integrity* than others in this same situation, and therefore has a higher risk for this problem. NANDA no longer recommends using this term.

Data. Pieces of information about health status (e.g., vital signs).

Objective Data. Information that you can clearly observe or measure, without need for someone to tell you (e.g., a pulse of 140 beats per minute). To remember this term, remember:

O-O = **O**bjective data are **O**bserved

---

[*] See Glossary for official definition of *Risk Nursing Diagnosis* published by NANDA (1994).

Subjective Data. Information the patient states or communicates; someone's perceptions. For example, "My heart feels like it's racing." To remember this term, remember:

S-S = **S**ubjective data are **S**tated (or communicated)

Cues. Synonymous with *data*.

Signs and Symptoms. Abnormal data that prompt you to suspect a health problem. *Signs* refer to objective data. *Symptoms* refer to subjective data.

Defining Characteristics. The signs and symptoms usually associated with a specific nursing diagnosis.

Data Base Assessment. Comprehensive data collection performed when someone first enters a health care facility to gain information about all aspects of health status.

Focus Assessment. Data collection that aims to gain specific (focused) information about only one aspect of health status.

Infer. To suspect something, or to attach meaning to a cue. For example, if an infant doesn't stop crying, no matter what's done for him, you might infer that *he's in pain*.

Inference. Something we suspect to be true, based on a logical conclusion. For example, the italicized words above.

Client-Centered (or Patient-Centered) Goal. A statement or phrase that details what the *patient or client* is expected to be able to do when the plan of care is terminated. For example, "Will be discharged home able to walk independently using a walker by 8/24."

Client-Centered Outcome. Synonymous with *client-centered goal*.

M-PCR. A mnemonic that stands for **M**onitor, **P**revent, **R**esolve, **C**ontrol: A plan of care should be designed to *monitor, prevent, resolve,* or *control* problems.

I. Practicing the Skill: Identifying Assumptions

Definition. Recognizing information taken for granted or presented as fact without evidence. For example, we might assume a woman on a maternity unit has just had a baby.

Why This Skill Promotes Critical Thinking

Critical thinking aims to make judgments based on evidence (fact). If we reason based on assumptions, our thinking may be flawed. By recognizing our assumptions, we can overcome our natural tendency to take things for granted, and get the *facts,* before going on to identify problems and make decisions.

Guidelines: How to Accomplish This Skill

The best way to identify assumptions is to *look* for them. Whenever making any important decisions, before you make a plan of action, ask questions like, "What's being taken for granted here?" and "How do I know that I've got the facts right?"

Practice Exercises: Skill I

1. Explain why the statement below is an assumption.

We've got to teach this patient how to stick to a low-salt diet because he eats whatever he wants even though his doctor told him not to eat salt.

2. What could happen if you planned nursing care based on the above assumption?
3. Read the following scenarios, then answer the questions that follow them.

■ Scenario One

Anita's plan today is to teach Jeff about diabetes. She's well prepared, and decides she'll create a positive attitude for Jeff by telling him about all the advances in diabetic care. She doesn't have much time, so she introduces herself, and starts telling him how much easier it is to manage diabetes than it used to be. She goes on to explain how easy it can be to learn the required diet, monitor blood sugar at home, and take insulin.

Jeff listens to all Anita has to say, asks a few questions, then leaves with his wife. As they drive off, he says to his wife in a discouraged tone, "She sure is a 'know-it-all,' isn't she?"

a. Based on the information provided above, what assumption does it seem Anita made about creating a positive attitude?
b. What key thing did Anita forget to do that might have helped her avoid making this assumption?
c. Why do you think Jeff said Anita was "a know-it-all"?

■ Scenario Two

Four-year-old Bobby is in the Emergency Department with his mother. He's fallen off his bike, and had an initial period of unconsciousness lasting about a minute. He's been examined, has no skull fracture, and is now awake and alert, ready to go home with his mother. The nurse gives his mother a computer print-out of instructions for checking Bobby's neurologic status at home, and says, "Let me know if you have questions."

a. What assumption does it seem the nurse has made?
b. What might happen if the nurse's assumption is incorrect?

■ **Scenario Three**

A friend of mine told me this story:

Years ago, I had just started working evenings in the Emergency Department of a seaside town hospital. We admitted a 54-year-old man, who I'll call Mr. Frank. Mr. Frank told me, "I just got here for vacation, and I'm not feeling so great. I had pneumonia at home, got treated, and thought I was better... but now my breathing feels lousy again." A check of his vital signs while he was sitting quietly revealed the following: T 99 P 138 R 36 BP 168/80.

As I helped him to the stretcher, he became significantly more short of breath. I checked his lung sounds and heard a lot of congestion. I notified the physician, and voiced my concern that Mr. Frank seemed quite ill. The doctor immediately examined him and ordered an EKG and chest x-ray.

During this time, we got very busy. I was helping another patient when the physician came to me and said, "I want you to give Mr. Frank 80 mg of furosemide (a diuretic) IV now, and discharge him."

I looked at him skeptically and said, *"Discharge* him?"

He said, "Yes. The waiting room is packed, we have no beds available in the hospital, and we need the stretcher. I'm sure the diuretic will help him get rid of this fluid."

Being new, and not really knowing this physician, I tried to tactfully voice my concern about this idea. "Can we give him some time to see how he responds?"

"Nope. This place is wild. I'm sending him home. He's going to a private physician in the morning. He'll be fine once he gets rid of some fluid. Discharge him with instructions to call if he doesn't feel better."

Reluctantly, I went to give Mr. Frank the furosemide. I still had trouble with the idea of sending this man home before knowing a response to the IV diuretic.

Then I decided to use my own clout as a nurse: I had established a rapport with the Franks, and they trusted me. Before I gave the drug, I said, "I realize the doctor has discharged you, but I'd be interested to see if there's any change in blood pressure after you get rid of some fluid. How would you feel about sitting in the waiting room, and I'll check your blood pressure in an hour?" Both the Franks thought this was a good idea, and went off to the waiting room. Only 45 minutes had passed, when there was a shout for help. I ran to the waiting room, and found Mr. Frank on the floor having a grand mal seizure. He then stopped breathing.

We were able to resuscitate Mr. Frank, and he was admitted to the hospital, diagnosed with electrolyte imbalance and heart failure, and discharged a week later.

a. What assumption does it seem the physician made about Mr. Frank's response to the furosemide?
b. Why do you think the nurse was so concerned about the assumption the physician made?
c. What assumption does it seem the nurse made about how the physician would respond to her if she cautioned him about discharging Mr. Frank?

II. Practicing the Skill: Identifying an Organized and Comprehensive Approach to Discovery (Assessment)

Definition. Choosing a systematic approach that enhances ability to discover all the information you need to fully understand the patient's health status.

Why This Skill Promotes Critical Thinking

One of the leading causes of critical thinking errors is making judgments or decisions based on incomplete information. If you have a well-thought-out, organized approach to assessment, you're more likely to notice when you've missed information than if you assess haphazardly. If you consistently use the same organized approach, you also form *habits* that help you be systematic and complete.

Guidelines: How to Accomplish This Skill

How you organize your assessment depends on the patient's health status:

- **If the person is acutely ill,** set immediate priorities by using an approach such as the ABC'S and MAA-U-AR approach listed in Display 3–7 (page 62).
- **If the person is generally healthy**, choose any organized method you find convenient. For example, use the head-to-toe approach, the body systems approach (Figure 3–2, page 52), the functional health patterns approach (Table 3–2, page 47), or follow a pre-printed assessment tool (page 105).
- **If the person has a specific problem,** begin by assessing *the problem* first, then go on to complete the assessment in the same way you would if the person were healthy.

Critical Thinking and Pre-printed Assessment Tools. Most facilities have developed assessment tools that nurses are required to complete for each patient. Some of these tools are designed for documentation of *data base assessment,* and others are designed for *focus assessment*. Pages 105–108 show an example of a data base assessment tool, and pages 109–110 show examples of focus assessment tools for neurologic and neurovascular assessment. If you'd like to see an example of what these assessment tools look like when they're completed by a nurse, check pages 156–161 in Appendix D.

While pre-printed assessment tools can help you develop habits that promote an organized and comprehensive approach to assessment, you must use these guides appropriately:

- Don't simply choose an assessment tool and follow it blindly, filling in the blanks: Before you begin using the tool, review it and determine why the information the tool guides you to collect is relevant. For example, if you're using the neurologic assessment tool on page 109, and you're collecting data about how the pupils react to light, find out why this information is relevant to determining neurologic status. Use critical thinking—make the connection between what information is collected and why it's relevant—to enhance your ability to perform a nursing assessment and move more quickly toward an expert level of thinking.

- Don't assume that once you've completed an assessment tool, you're finished with your assessment. Patient situations vary: Use critical thinking strategies like reviewing your completed assessment tool and asking yourself questions such as, "What else should I be looking for?" and "What could I have missed?"
- Remember the importance of gathering both subjective data (patient's perceptions) and objective data (your observations).
- Keep in mind that assessment tools don't prompt you to use all your resources: Once you've interviewed and examined your patient, ask yourself, "What other resources might provide additional information about this person's health status (medical and nursing records, significant others, other health care professionals)?"

To help you become skilled at identifying an organized and comprehensive approach to assessment:

1. Choose a method of assessment and use it consistently.
2. Locate assessment tools that are designed for your patient's specific situation, and practice using them.
3. Keep in mind that a body systems approach to assessment helps you collect data about *medical problems*. Nursing models, such as functional health patterns, help you collect data about *human responses* to medical problems or changes in life.

Practice Exercises: Skill II

1. You're working as a school nurse and have been asked to screen the students for possible medical problems before they see the doctor. Identify an organized, comprehensive approach to assessing for signs and symptoms of a medical problem.
2. You're working in community health and are making a home visit to Mrs. Schmidt, who has a newborn child and seven other children under 12 years old. Both the baby and the mother are healthy. Identify an organized and comprehensive approach to assessing for problems with human responses.
3. Read the following scenarios, then answer the questions that follow them.

■ Scenario One

Pearl is an 89-year-old grandmother who is admitted overnight after fracturing her left ankle. She had surgery and a cast applied today. The cast goes from her toes to below the knee. Her toes are visible, and she can wiggle them freely. A small window has been cut in the cast over the dorsalis pedis pulse. Routine hospital protocols state that anyone with a new cast must have neurovascular checks every 2 hours for the first day of hospitalization.

You know the following acrostic helps you remember the things you need to check when performing a neurovascular assessment for someone with a cast:

Maggie **C**hewed **N**uts **E**very **P**lace **S**he **W**ent stands for:

Movement, **C**olor, **N**umbness, **E**dema, **P**ulses, **S**ensation, **W**armth

a. Using the above acrostic to help you assess systematically, how would you assess to determine the neurovascular status of Pearl's injured leg?
b. Why is it necessary to monitor each of the above assessment parameters to determine neurovascular status?
c. What would you do if Pearl told you her toes felt numb and cold?

■ Scenario Two

You're about to give Mr. Wu digoxin by mouth. You know that the mnemonic TACT helps you remember what you need to assess to monitor responses to medications and determine whether there are any reasons to withhold them:

T = Therapeutic effect (is there a *therapeutic effect?*)

A = Adverse reactions (are there signs of *adverse reactions?*)

C = Contraindications (are there any *contraindications* to giving this drug?)

T = Toxicity/overdose (are there signs of *toxicity or overdose?*)

Using TACT to focus your assessment to systematically gather information about how Mr. Wu is responding to the digoxin:

a. How would you assess him to decide whether to give the digoxin?
b. Why is it important to determine all of the things listed in the mnemonic TACT?

■ Scenario Three

You've just admitted Gerome, who fell off his bike, hit his head, and had a short period of unconsciousness. He is now awake and alert, but is admitted for 24 hours of neurologic monitoring. The physician orders neurologic assessments every hour. The neurologic focus assessment tool your hospital uses provides these key terms to guide you to collect and record the following information:

Vital Signs

Temp.   Pulse   Resp.   BP

Eye Opening

Spontaneous   To command   To pain   No response

Best Motor Response

Obeys commands   Localizes pain   Flexion withdrawal
Abnormal flexion   Abnormal Extension   No response

Best Verbal Response

Oriented   Confused   Inappropriate words
Incomprehensible words   No response

Pupillary Reaction

Right eye: Size of pupil   Reaction to light (brisk, sluggish)

Left eye: Size of pupil   Reaction to light (brisk, sluggish)

Purposeful Limb Movement

Circle words that best describe limb movement below:

Right arm:

Spontaneous   To command   Paralysis

Visible muscle contraction; no movement

Weak contraction; not enough to overcome gravity

Moves against gravity, not to external resistance

Normal range of motion; can be overcome by increased gravity

Normal muscle strength

Right leg:

Spontaneous   To command   Paralysis

Visible muscle contraction; no movement

Weak contraction; not enough to overcome gravity

Moves against gravity, not to external resistance

Normal range of motion; can be overcome by increased gravity

Normal muscle strength

Left arm:

Spontaneous   To command   Paralysis

Visible muscle contraction; no movement

Weak contraction; not enough to overcome gravity

Moves against gravity, not to external resistance

Normal range of motion; can be overcome by increased gravity

Normal muscle strength

Left leg:

Spontaneous   To command   Paralysis

Visible muscle contraction; no movement

Weak contraction; not enough to overcome gravity

Moves against gravity, not to external resistance

Normal range of motion; can be overcome by increased gravity

Normal muscle strength

Limb Sensation

Prick limb with sterile needle:

Right arm:	Normal	Decreased	Absent
Right leg:	Normal	Decreased	Absent
Left arm:	Normal	Decreased	Absent
Left leg:	Normal	Decreased	Absent

Seizure Activity

Describe seizures in nurse's notes.

Gag Reflex

Present   Absent

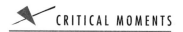 CRITICAL MOMENTS

When identifying inconsistencies, what you *don't* see or hear may be more important than what you *do* see or hear. Ask yourself, "What would I expect to see, given this situation?" and "Why don't I see it?"

Consider Scenario Three (page 101), then answer the following questions:

a. How would you assess Gerome to determine the status of each of the neurologic assessment parameters beginning on page 102?
b. Why are the above data relevant to determining neurologic status?
c. What would you do if, on admission, Gerome demonstrated normal neurologic assessment findings, but 2 hours later he is more difficult to arouse (he awakens only if you shake him and call his name)?
d. What would you do if one pupil started to become more sluggish in its response to light than the other?
e. What would you do if you noted a general pattern of the pulse getting slower than baseline pulse?

OTHER PERSPECTIVES

The best way to find the best answer is to find a lot of answers.

OTHER PERSPECTIVES

Often, it takes just one nurse to implement a new idea, and with any luck you may have an epidemic on your hands.
Anne Parrish (1994).

CRITICAL MOMENTS

If a little knowledge is dangerous, there are a lot of dangerous people walking around out there. Don't just assume others know more than you do, even if they sound knowledgeable: Ask questions, seek clarification, and think independently (e.g., Ask, "Where might I find a reference to add to my knowledge of this?").

CRITICAL MOMENTS

Pilots have a "sterile cockpit." During a specific period of time before landing and after takeoff, no one is to enter the cockpit, and cockpit conversation is limited to flight procedures only. To ensure that this is so, pilots' conversations are recorded. Nurses can learn from pilots. During crucial moments, like preparing medications, ask not to be disturbed, and don't disturb others.

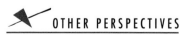

OTHER PERSPECTIVES

There are no learning disabilities—only differences.

NURSING ADMISSION ASSESSMENT

DATE _____ TIME OF ARRIVAL _____

FROM _____

ACCOMPANIED BY _____

VIA: WHEELCHAIR _____ STRETCHER _____ AMBULATORY _____

ID BRACELET _____ INFORMATION OBTAINED FROM _____

I. VITAL STATISTICS

PROSTHESIS, APPLIANCES OR OTHER DEVICES:

TEMP _____ PULSE _____ RESP _____

ORAL _____ RECTAL _____ AXILLARY _____

BP _____ RA _____ LA _____ POSITION _____

WEIGHT _____ HEIGHT _____

SCALE: BED _____ CHAIR _____ STANDING _____

DEFERRED _____

ORIENTED TO ROOM _____

DENTURES _____   *WALKER/CANE/CRUTCHES __

FULL: UPPER _____ LOWER_____   *ARTIFICIAL LIMBS _____

PARTIAL: UPPER _____ LOWER _____   *BRACES _____

EYE GLASSES _____   *FALSE EYE _____

CONTACT LENSES _____   WIG _____

HEARING AID _____

OTHER _____

COMMENTS _____

PATIENT HAS BROUGHT TO HOSPITAL? YES _____ NO _____

EXCEPTIONS _____

II. ALLERGIES: DRUGS _____ DYES _____ FOOD _____ OTHER _____ NONE KNOWN _____

SPECIFY AGENT	DESCRIBE REACTION (IF KNOWN)

III. HEALTH PERCEPTION-HEALTH MAINTENANCE

A. PRESENT ILLNESS:

1. ADMITTING DIAGNOSIS _____

2. REASON FOR ADMISSION (PATIENT'S STATEMENT) _____

3. DURATION OF PRESENT ILLNESS_____

4. PAST AND PRESENT TREATMENT OF PRESENT ILLNESS AND RESPONSE_____

5. PATIENT AWARE OF DIAGNOSIS: YES _____ NO _____ NOT ESTABLISHED _____

B. PREVIOUS ILLNESSES: (INCLUDING HOSPITALIZATION)

_____

_____

8183 PG 1 (REV 9/90)

Figure 5–1

Assessment tools are reprinted with permission of the Bryn Mawr Hospital, Bryn Mawr, PA.

C. ARE YOU TAKING ANY MEDICATIONS (PRESCRIBED OR OVER THE COUNTER) YES _____ NO _____

MEDICATION	DOSE	WHEN DO YOU TAKE IT	WHY DO YOU TAKE IT	LAST DOSE	BROUGHT TO HOSPITAL		DISPOSITION
					YES	NO	

D. DO YOU OR HAVE YOU EVER USED?

	YES	NO	LAST USED	FREQUENCY/AMOUNT
ALCOHOL				
RECREATIONAL DRUGS				

E. DO YOU SMOKE? YES _____ PKS/DAY _____ HOW LONG _____

    NO: DID YOU EVER SMOKE? NO ____ YES ____ PKS/DAY _____ HOW LONG _____ WHEN DID YOU QUIT _____

IV. COGNITIVE PERCEPTUAL: HEADACHE _____ SEIZURES _____ BLACKOUTS _____ DIZZINESS _____ NO C/O _____

A. LEVEL OF CONSCIOUSNESS: ALERT _____ DROWSY _____ RESPONDS TO: PAIN _____ VERBAL STIMULI _____ UNRESPONSIVE _____

B. ORIENTED: TIME _____ PLACE _____ PERSON _____ COMMENTS _____

C. MOOD: RELAXED _____ ANXIOUS _____ SAD _____ ANGRY _____ WITHDRAWN _____ OTHER_____

D. RECENT MEMORY CHANGE: YES _____ NO _____ SPECIFY_____

E. RESPONDS TO DIRECTIONS: YES _____ NO _____ SPECIFY_____

F. SPEECH: CLEAR _____ SLURRED _____ GARBLED _____ UNABLE TO SPEAK _____ APHASIC_____

G. LANGUAGE SPOKEN: ENGLISH _____ OTHER _____

H. HEARING: WNL _____ IMPAIRED _____ CORRECTED _____ DEAF _____ SIGN LANGUAGE _____ LIP READS _____

I. VISION: WNL _____ IMPAIRED _____ CORRECTED _____ BLIND _____

J. PAIN: YES _____ NO _____ DESCRIBE _____

    HOW DO YOU MANAGE YOUR PAIN? _____

K. LEARNING READINESS: NO LIMITATIONS _____ WILLING TO LEARN _____ RESISTS LEARNING _____

    EMOTIONALLY READY TO LEARN: YES _____ NO _____ REQUIRES CONCRETE LANGUAGE/REINFORCEMENT _____ FORGETFUL _____

    TEACHING TO BE DIRECTED PRIMARILY TO _____
                            FAMILY MEMBER/SIGNIFICANT OTHER

L. COMMENTS_____

V. ROLE RELATIONSHIP (PSYCHOSOCIAL) / DISCHARGE PLANNING

A. OCCUPATION _____

B. LIVE ALONE _____ WITH FAMILY _____ NURSING HOME _____ OTHER _____ COMMENT _____

C. DESCRIBE PHYSICAL ENVIRONMENT_____

D. ANTICIPATED DISCHARGE TO: ECF _____ HOME CARE SERVICES _____

    OTHER _____ HOME _____ IF GOING HOME, WHO COULD HELP YOU WITH

    HEALTHCARE NEEDS AFTER DISCHARGE?_____

E. DO YOU WISH TO SEE A MEMBER OF THE CLERGY WHILE YOU ARE HERE? YES _____ NO _____ AFFILIATION_____

F. COMMENTS_____

VI. HEALTH HISTORY/ASSESSMENT

A. CARDIOVASCULAR: ANGINA _____ ARRHYTHMIA _____ MURMUR _____ EDEMA _____ PALPITATIONS _____

    CHEST PAIN _____ MI _____ CVA _____ ANEURYSM _____ HYPERTENSION _____

    PACEMAKER _____ TYPE _____ NO C/O _____

    PULSE: STRONG _____ WEAK _____ REGULAR _____ IRREGULAR _____

    RIGHT DORSALIS PEDAL PULSE: STRONG _____ WEAK _____ ABSENT _____

    LEFT DORSALIS PEDAL PULSE: STRONG _____ WEAK _____ ABSENT _____

    COMMENTS_____

Figure 5–1 *Continued*

B. RESPIRATORY: COUGH _____ PRODUCTIVE _____ PAIN _____ DESCRIBE _____

FREQUENT COLDS _____ HOARSENESS _____ ASTHMA _____ TB _____ SOB: ON EXERTION _____ AT REST _____ NO C/O _____

COMMENTS _____

_____

C. RENAL: KIDNEY STONES _____ INFECTIONS _____ RETENTION _____ BURNING _____ POLYURIA _____ DYSURIA _____ NO C/O _____

URINARY DEVICES? _____ TYPE _____

INCONTINENCE _____ DAYTME _____ NOCTURNAL _____ STRESS _____

DO YOU GET UP DURING NIGHT TO URINATE? YES _____ NO _____

COMMENTS _____

_____

D. GASTROINTESTINAL (NUTRITION/METABOLIC)

1. HISTORY OF DIABETES? YES _____ NO _____ DO YOU TEST FOR SUGAR? YES _____ NO _____ URINE _____ BLOOD _____

DIET CONTROLLED _____ INSULIN DEPENDENT _____ ORAL HYPOGLYCEMICS _____

NUMBER OF YEARS _____ PREVIOUS DIABETES EDUCATION: YES _____ NO _____

2. NUMBER OF MEALS/DAY _____ SNACKS _____ SPECIAL DIET _____

3. PATIENT'S ABILITY TO EAT: INDEPENDENT _____ WITH ASSISTANCE _____ SPECIFY _____

DIFFICULTY SWALLOWING _____

4. WEIGHT CHANGE IN THE LAST SIX MONTHS: NONE _____ LOST _____ LBS GAINED _____ LBS

5. DO YOU EXPERIENCE NAUSEA/VOMITING? YES _____ NO _____ RELATED TO _____

6. DO YOU EXPERIENCE CRAMPING _____ HEARTBURN _____ RECTAL PAIN _____ GAS _____ LAST BM: _____

7. BOWEL: USUAL TIME: _____ A.M. _____ P.M. FREQUENCY: DAILY _____ EVERY OTHER DAY _____ OTHER _____

INCONTINENCE _____ DEVICES USED _____

COLOR: BROWN _____ CLAY-COLORED _____ BLACK _____ BLOOD _____

CONSTIPATION: NONE _____ OCCASIONALLY _____ FREQUENTY _____

DIARRHEA: NONE _____ OCCASIONALLY _____ FREQUENTLY _____ OSTOMY _____

LAXATIVES/ENEMAS USED/HOW OFTEN? (SPECIFY) _____

8. ABDOMEN: SOFT _____ NON-TENDER _____ NON-DISTENDED _____ FIRM _____ TENDER _____ DISTENDED _____

BOWEL SOUNDS: PRESENT _____ ABSENT _____

COMMENTS: _____

_____

E. SKIN CONDITION

COLOR: WNL _____ PALE _____ CYANOTIC _____ JAUNDICE _____ OTHER _____

TEMP: WARM _____ COOL _____ TURGOR: WNL _____ POOR _____

EDEMA: NO _____ YES _____ DESCRIPTION/LOCATION _____

LESIONS: NO _____ YES _____ DESCRIPTION/LOCATION _____

DECUBITUS: NO _____ YES _____ LOCATION(S) _____ (SEE TISSUE TRAUMA FORM)

BRUISES: NO _____ YES _____ DESCRIPTION/LOCATION _____

RASHES: NO _____ YES _____ DESCRIPTION/LOCATION _____

REDNESS: NO _____ YES _____ DESCRIPTION/LOCATION _____

COMMENTS: _____

_____

Figure 5–1   *Continued*

F. MUSCULO-SKELETAL: CRAMPING _____ ARTHRITIS _____ STIFFNESS _____ SWELLING _____ NO C/O _____

MOTOR FUNCTION: RIGHT ARM: WNL ____ AMPUTATED ____ SPASTIC ____ FLACCID ____ WEAKNESS ____ PARALYSIS ____ OTHER ____

LEFT ARM: WNL ____ AMPUTATED ____ SPASTIC ____ FLACCID ____ WEAKNESS ____ PARALYSIS ____ OTHER ____

RIGHT LEG: WNL ____ AMPUTATED ____ SPASTIC ____ FLACCID ____ WEAKNESS ____ PARALYSIS ____ OTHER ____

LEFT LEG: WNL ____ AMPUTATED ____ SPASTIC ____ FLACCID ____ WEAKNESS ____ PARALYSIS ____ OTHER ____

COMMENTS _____

_____

VII. SLEEP-REST/ACTIVITY

A. USUAL SLEEP PATTERN: BEDTIME _____ HOURS SLEPT _____ NAPS: NO _____ YES _____

B. DIFFICULTY FALLING ASLEEP: NO _____ YES _____ SPECIFY _____

C. SLEEP AIDS USED: NO _____ YES _____ SPECIFY _____

D. DOES PATIENT HAVE DIFFICULTY/PROBLEMS IN:

BATHING: NO _____ YES _____ SPECIFY _____

DRESSING: NO _____ YES _____ SPECIFY _____

AMBULATING: NO _____ YES _____ BALANCE/GAIT: STEADY _____ UNSTEADY _____ TIRES EASILY _____ WEAKNESS _____

COMMENTS _____

VIII. SEXUAL HEALTH (FEMALES)

A. LMP _____ LAST PAP SMEAR _____

B. DO YOU EXAMINE YOUR BREASTS? YES _____ NO _____ HOW OFTEN? _____

C. IF NO, DO YOU KNOW HOW? YES _____ NO _____ WOULD YOU BE INTERESTED IN LEARNING? YES _____ NO _____

PAMPHLET GIVEN? YES _____ NO _____ COMMENTS _____

IX. ASSESSMENT SUMMARY: _____

_____

_____

X. NURSING DIAGNOSES: _____

_____

_____

_____

_____

XI. THE FOLLOWING SECTIONS WERE DEFERRED ON ADMISSION (IDENTIFY BY SECTION NUMBER): _____

_____

REASON: _____

DATE/TIME	COMPLETED BY	PRIMARY NURSE	DATE/TIME	REVIEWED BY PRIMARY NURSE
_____/_____	_____ RN	YES ____ NO ____	_____/_____	_____ RN
_____/_____	_____ RN	YES ____ NO ____	_____/_____	_____ RN

8183 PG 4 (REV 9/90)

Figure 5–1 *Continued*

**THE BRYN MAWR HOSPITAL
NURSING DEPARTMENT**

NEUROLOGICAL ASSESSMENT SHEET

1MM · 2MM · 3MM · 4MM · 5MM · 6MM · 7MM · 8MM · 9MM

	DATE												
	TIME												
V I T A L S	BLOOD PRESSURE											RESPIRATORY TYPE	
	PULSE											N = NORMAL	
	TEMPERATURE											CS = CHEYNE STOKES	
	RESPIRATORY RATE											SH = SUSTAINED HYPERVENTILATION	
	RESPIRATORY TYPE												

COMA SCALE

EYES OPEN	SPONTANEOUSLY	4										E = EYES CLOSED BY SWELLING
	TO COMMAND	3										
	TO PAIN	2										
	NO RESPONSE	1										
BEST MOTOR RESPONSE	OBEYS COMMANDS	6										
	LOCALIZES PAIN	5										RECORD BEST ARM RESPONSE
	FLEXION WITHDRAWAL	4										
	FLEXION (ABNORMAL)	3										
	EXTENSION (ABNORMAL)	2										
	NO RESPONSE	1										
BEST VERBAL RESPONSE	ORIENTED	5										T = ENDOTRACHEAL TUBE OR TRACHEOSTOMY
	CONFUSED	4										
	INAPPROPRIATE WORDS	3										
	INCOMPREHENSIBLE SOUNDS	2										A = APHASIA
	NO RESPONSE	1										
TOTAL SCORE												

PUPILS

SIZE	R											B = BRISK · S = SLUGGISH · N = NO REACTION · C = CLOSED
REACTION												
SIZE	L											SC = SUSTAINED CONSTRICTION 2° CATARACT SURGERY
REACTION												

LIMB MOVEMENT / LIMB SENSATION

GRADE LIMB SPONTANEOUS OR TO COMMAND. DO NOT RATE REFLEX MOVEMENT	RA											LIMB MOVEMENT SCALE
	RL											0 = PARALYSIS
	LA											1 = VISIBLE MUSCLE CONTRACTION; NO MOVEMENT
	LL											2 = WEAK CONTRACTION; NOT ENOUGH TO OVERCOME GRAVITY
DULL	RA											3 = MOVE AGAINST GRAVITY; NOT EXTERNAL RESISTANCE
	RL											4 = NORMAL ROM; CAN BE OVERCOME BY INCREASED GRAVITY
	LA											5 = NORMAL MUSCLE STRENGTH
	LL											SENSATION CODES
SHARP	RA											N = NORMAL
	RL											D = DECREASED
	LA											A = ABSENT
	LL											
SEIZURE ACTIVITY												A = ABSENT · P = PRESENT
GAG REFLEX												A = ABSENT · P = PRESENT
INITIALS												

SIGNATURE	INITIALS	SIGNATURE	INITIALS

F8084
(REV 1/91)

Figure 5–2

Assessment tools are reprinted with permission of the Bryn Mawr Hospital, Bryn Mawr, PA.

THE BRYN MAWR HOSPITAL
NURSING SERVICE

NEURO-VASCULAR ASSESSMENT FLOW SHEET

EXTREMITY(IES) TO BE ASSESSED:

FREQUENCY OF ASSESSMENT:

TYPE OF EXTERNAL SUPPORT:

Date	Time	Hospital Day / Post-Op Day	Limb	Color	Capillary Refill	Temp.	Edema	Sensation	Numbness & Tingling	Motion	Pulse	Proprioception	Comments	Signature

FORM 8066

KEY

Limb(s): Specify RUE, LUE, RLE, LLE
Color: Pink, Pale, Cyanotic
Capillary Refill: Rapid, Slow
Temperature: Warm, Cool, Cold
Edema: Absent (A), Present(P)
Sensation: Absent (A), Decreased (D), Present (P)

Numbness (N), Tingling (T): Present (P), Decreased (D), Absent (A)
Motion: Present (P), Decreased (D), Absent (A)
Pulses: Present (P), Absent (A)
Proprioception: Present (P), Absent (A)
NA: Not Applicable
*: See Nurses Notes

Figure 5-3

Assessment tools are reprinted with permission of the Bryn Mawr Hospital, Bryn Mawr, PA.

III. Practicing the Skill: Checking Accuracy and Reliability of Data (Validation)

Definition. Verifying information to determine if it's factual.

Why This Skill Promotes Critical Thinking

As previously stated, critical thinking aims to make judgments based on evidence (fact). Without checking whether your information is accurate and factual, you may make decisions based on incorrect information. Since validating (verifying) your information requires you to gather more information (see Guidelines: How to Accomplish This Skill *below*), it also promotes comprehensive data collection (Skill II).

Guidelines: How to Accomplish This Skill

To check accuracy and reliability, review the data already gathered and ask, "What data might need verifying here?" Then focus your assessment to gain more information to verify or negate that information. For example, an elderly person may have told you that she took her medicine. To verify this, interview significant others or caregivers, or check previous records.

Practice Exercises: Skill III

For each of the following, determine how you would validate whether the data are accurate and reliable:

1. The off-going nurse tells you that your patient is depressed and angry about being in the hospital.
2. Your patient tells you he thinks his blood sugar was about 104 when he tested it a half an hour ago.
3. You take a blood pressure in your patient's left arm and find it to be abnormally high.
4. Your patient's care plan states that he has *Knowledge Deficit: Diabetic Foot Care as evidenced by frequent foot ulcers.*

IV. Practicing the Skill: Distinguishing Normal from Abnormal and Identifying Signs and Symptoms

Definition. Determining what data are *within* normal range and what data are *outside* the usual range for normalcy. Data that are abnormal are considered a sign, symptom, or cue of a possible problem. For example, if a 58-year-old man has a pulse of 46 beats per minute, you know that this is *abnormal*. You may consider it to be a sign of possible cardiac problems, because a normal pulse rate rarely drops below 60 beats per minute in someone this age (healthy young athletes sometimes have pulses as slow as 46).

Why This Skill Promotes Critical Thinking

Recognizing abnormal data (signs and symptoms) is the first step to problem identification: Signs and symptoms are like "red flags" that prompt you to suspect a health problem. If you miss "red flags," you miss recognizing problems.

Guidelines: How to Accomplish This Skill

To identify signs and symptoms, use your senses (sight, hearing, touch, and smell) to gain all the relevant information. For example, if you *see* cloudy urine, you *smell* it to check its odor.

Ask the following questions:

1. **How do my patient's data compare with accepted standards for normalcy for someone of this age, culture, disease process, and lifestyle?** If the person's data aren't within normal accepted standards, they are abnormal, and considered a possible sign or symptom of a problem.
2. **How do my patient's *current data* compare with the *previously collected data*?** This question is especially helpful in situations where the patient has chronic signs and symptoms, and you're trying to decide whether the signs and symptoms are getting worse. For example, an asthmatic may always be slightly wheezy. However, if this same person now is more wheezy than *before,* consider this increased wheeziness to be a sign of increasing problems.

Practice Exercises: Skill IV

1. Place an "S" next to the data below that either are signs or symptoms of a possible problem, or signs or symptoms of a problem that's getting worse. Place an "O" if it's neither a sign nor a symptom. Place a question mark if you need more information to decide.
   a. ____ Temperature of 99.6.
   b. ____ Bilateral pulmonary rales.
   c. ____ Someone tells you they rarely sleep more than 3 hours at a time.
   d. ____ Someone's nasogastric drainage has turned from brown to red.
   e. ____ Someone's abdominal incision is slightly red around the sutures.
   f. ____ A 2-year-old is inconsolable when his mother leaves the room.
   g. ____ Someone with no health problems has developed ankle edema.
   h. ____ Someone tells you they bathe every other week.
   i. ____ Someone on kidney dialysis never urinates.
   j. ____ Pulse of 56 per minute.

2. For each question mark you placed above, explain *what else* you'd want to know before you decided whether the information is a sign or a symptom.

V. Practicing the Skill: Making Inferences (Drawing Valid Conclusions)

Definition. Making deductions that follow logically by interpreting subjective and objective data. For example, note the data on the left below with the corresponding inferences on the right.

Data (Cues)	Inference
Frowning	Seems worried
White blood cell count = 14,000	Probable infection
Deaf	Has communication problems

Why This Skill Promotes Critical Thinking

Your ability to interpret data and draw conclusions (make inferences) is essential to getting a beginning understanding of the problems. It helps you focus your assessment to look for *other information* that might support or negate your inferences. For example, if you infer that an elevated white blood cell count may indicate an infection, you know to look for signs and symptoms of infection.

Guidelines: How to Accomplish This Skill

Ability to make correct inferences requires problem-specific knowledge and knowledge of cultural influences. For example, to make the inference of *probable infection,* you need to know what a normal white blood cell count is, *and* that an elevated white blood cell count is a sign of infection. Your knowledge of cultural influences is essential to making inferences about psychosocial data. For example, you may infer that someone's lack of eye contact indicates that he is mistrustful if you aren't aware that in his culture, lack of eye contact indicates respect.

To improve your ability to make correct inferences:

- Avoid making inferences based on only one cue.
- Once you've made an inference, verify whether it's correct by gathering more information.

To form habits that help you avoid jumping to conclusions, begin your statements about inferences by saying, "*I suspect this information indicates*...." Using this phrase reinforces that inferences are *suspicions* that guide you to collect more data to decide if your suspicions are correct. Once you're *sure* your inference is correct, you can begin to view it as *fact.*

Practice Exercises: Skill V

1. Make an inference about each of the following data (begin your inference by writing, "I suspect this information indicates....").
   a. Temperature of 102° F for 3 days.
   b. A mother tells you she can't afford prenatal care.
   c. A diabetic is 100 pounds overweight and says his blood sugar is always out of control, even though he watches his food intake and takes his insulin regularly.
   d. A 5-year-old child whose mother told you he broke his leg falling down the stairs keeps looking at his mother before answering any of your questions.
   e. A grandmother who usually is alert and active in her church presents with an unkempt appearance and seems a bit confused.

VI. Practicing the Skill: Clustering Related Cues (Data)

Definition. Grouping data in such a way that it helps you see relationships among the data. For example, you may have grouped the following cues together:

Two years old, temperature 100, pulse 144 per minute, rash all over trunk, recent measles exposure, never had measles, screaming that he wants his mother.

If you consider the relationship among the above data, you may suspect that the child's rapid pulse is related to his screaming, rather than a sign of cardiac problems. If you consider all of the above data, *you'll probably suspect these symptoms indicate the child may have measles.*

Why This Skill Promotes Critical Thinking

Grouping information together applies the scientific principle of classifying information to enhance ability to see relationships between and among data. When you group related information together, it helps you determine whether there *are relationships* among the data. It also helps you get a beginning picture of patterns of health or illness.

Guidelines: How to Accomplish This Skill

How you cluster data depends on your purpose:

- If your goal is to determine the status of medical problems or physiologic responses, cluster the data according to body systems (see Fig. 3–2, page 52).
- If your goal is to determine human responses, cluster the data according to a nursing model (e.g., see Tables 3–2 and 3–3 on pages 47–48).

Practice Exercises: Skill VI

Read the following scenarios, then answer the questions that follow them.

▪ Scenario One

The 16-year-old baby sitter next door calls and tells you that Jackson, the 7-year-old she's watching, was stung by a bee on the ear an hour ago. She tells you the ear is swollen, and asks if you'll come and check him to decide whether he needs to go to the hospital. You go over, and examine the child. He asks you if he might die "like the kid on *911* almost did." The baby sitter tells you she's afraid because she doesn't know where the mother is. You check the ear and find it red, swollen, and free of the stinger. When asked, Jackson tells you he was stung before, but that wasn't as scary. Jackson has no rash and no wheezing. He asks if he could have a popsicle and watch TV. His pulse and respirations are normal.

a. Cluster the available information that will help you determine Jackson's physical health status.
b. Cluster the available information that will help you determine Jackson's human responses.
c. Cluster the available information that will help you determine the baby sitter's learning needs.

▪ Scenario Two

It's 11 A.M., and you've just admitted Mr. Nelson, a 41-year-old businessman who has acute abdominal pain. He's never been in the hospital and tells you he hates everything about hospitals. He's been vomiting for 2 days, and unable to keep any food down. His abdomen is distended, and he has no bowel sounds. He is scheduled to go to the operating room at 2 P.M for emergency exploratory surgery. He's telling you he's worried because his brother died in the hospital after a car accident, when suddenly he doubles over and says, "Oh God, this is really getting worse!" You take his vital signs, and they are as follows: T 101 P 132 R 32 BP 140/80. These signs are the same as those taken an hour ago, except that before, his pulse was 104.

a. Cluster available information that will help you determine Mr. Nelson's physical status.
b. Cluster available information that will help you determine Mr. Nelson's human responses.

VII. Practicing the Skill: Distinguishing Relevant from Irrelevant

Definition. Deciding what information is pertinent to understanding the situations at hand and what information is immaterial.

Why This Skill Promotes Critical Thinking

When faced with a lot of information, narrowing it down to *only the facts that are pertinent* prevents your brain from being cluttered with *unnecessary* facts. Deciding what's relevant is also an example of one of the principles of the scientific method: classifying or categorizing information into groups of related (relevant) information.

Guidelines: How to Accomplish This Skill

This skill is especially difficult for novices. They tend to find themselves asking, "How can I decide what's relevant, if I don't know very much about the *problems* yet?" It *does* require problem-specific knowledge to decide what's relevant. For instance, if you have a patient with a heart problem, you need to know the common causes and usual progression of heart problems to decide what information is relevant (e.g., if you know that *ankle edema* is an early sign of congestive heart failure, you recognize it as being a *relevant sign* to consider when determining cardiac status).

Here are some strategies that can help you determine what's relevant, even with limited knowledge:

1. List the abnormal data collected.
2. Then ask yourself, "Could there be any connection between this (abnormal data) and that (abnormal data)?"
3. As appropriate, ask the person or significant others, "Do you think there's any relationship between this (abnormal data) and that (abnormal data)?"
4. Data that might be connected to other data are likely to be relevant to getting a beginning understanding of the problems.
5. To decide specifically if a piece of information is relevant to a problem, compare the person's signs, symptoms, and risk factors with the signs, symptoms, and risk factors of the problem you suspect. For example, if the person has no support systems and you suspect *Ineffective Coping*, you'd consider "no support systems" as being relevant to the *Ineffective Coping* because "lack of support systems" is a risk factor for *Ineffective Coping*.

Practice Exercises: Skill VII

Consider the following scenarios. Then answer the questions that follow them.

■ Scenario One

You're working in community health, and are making a weekly visit to Mrs. Blondell, who is 80 years old and had a cerebrovascular accident (CVA) a month ago. Today you notice she seems to be increasingly confused: She knows where she is, but forgets what day it is and doesn't seem to remember her daily routine.

1. You know that confusion in the elderly can be caused by any of the following: medications, infection, decreased oxygen to the brain, electrolyte imbalance, brain pathology. You assess Mrs. Blondell and gather the data listed below. Consider each piece of information below, and decide its possible relevance to the problem of confusion: List whether you think it's relevant and why.
   a. Recently started taking buspirone hydrochloride for anxiety
   b. Temperature: 100° F orally
   c. History of a myocardial infarction 5 years ago
   d. Seems dehydrated
   e. Has no allergies
   f. Regular diet

■ Scenario Two

You assess Mrs. Clark, a 32-year-old diabetic. She's come in for a routine visit. When you ask how the new diet is going, she breaks down into tears, saying, "I'm *never* going to be able to do this!"

1. Consider each piece of information below, and decide its possible relevance to the problem with sticking to the diabetic diet: List whether you think it's relevant and why.
   a. Diagnosed with diabetes 2 months ago
   b. Vital signs within normal limits
   c. Complains of constipation
   d. Married with three school age children
   e. Loves to cook
   f. Has always been 50 pounds overweight
   g. Allergic to aspirin

VIII. Practicing the Skill: Recognizing Inconsistencies

Definition. Realizing when health assessment data present conflicting information. For example, suppose you have someone who tells you he has no pain after chest surgery. However, he moves very little, guards his chest carefully, and barely breathes when you ask him to take a deep breath. The way this person is moving is inconsistent with his statements of being pain-free.

Why This Skill Promotes Critical Thinking

Recognizing inconsistencies prompts you to investigate issues more closely. It helps you focus your assessment to gain the additional information you need to better understand the problem. For example, in the above case, you might say, "It seems to me that you aren't moving very well. I suspect you're having more pain that you admit. I want you to be comfortable, so that you move well and are able to take deep breaths to clear your lungs. Are you sure there isn't a particular spot that's causing you discomfort?"

Guidelines: How to Accomplish This Skill

One way to recognize inconsistencies is to compare what the patient *states* (subjective data) with what you *observe* (objective data). If what the person *states isn't* supported by what you *observe,* as in the above example, you've identified inconsistent information and need to investigate further.

As with most of these skills, recognizing inconsistencies requires a problem-specific knowledge. For example: Suppose your neighbor tells you, "I've been staying in bed because I must have strained my back...it's been aching on the right side." On further questioning, she says she also has a fever and cloudy urine. What would you suspect? If you're knowledgeable about how back injuries present, you'd recognize that the symptoms are *inconsistent* with a back injury, and more consistent with a kidney infection.

Recognizing this inconsistency would prompt you to urge her to get medical treatment, rather than simply rest in bed.

To recognize these types of inconsistencies with limited knowledge:

- Determine the signs and symptoms of the problem you suspect (or your patient has identified) by looking up the problem in a reference (e.g., if you suspect pneumonia, look up the signs and symptoms of pneumonia in a textbook).
- Then compare the information in the reference with your patient's data. If your patient's signs and symptoms are *different* from those listed in the reference, you've identified inconsistencies, and must investigate further: Assess the person more closely, and consider other problems that the signs and symptoms might represent.

Practice Exercises: Skill VIII

Read the following scenarios, then answer the questions that follow them.

■ Scenario One

You're interviewing Cathy in the prenatal clinic, 2 weeks before delivery. You ask her how she feels about the baby coming. She tells you she's happy that she'll get to see it in only 2 weeks. When you ask her if she has any questions about the delivery, she tells you she's been going to birthing classes with her boyfriend, and feels like she knows what to expect.

You review her records and notice that her first clinic visit was 2 weeks ago, when she came with her mother.

a. Identify inconsistencies in the above scenario.
b. Explain what you might do to clarify the inconsistencies you identified above.

◼ Scenario Two

You're in the grocery store, and a woman who appears to be about 20 years old comes up to you and says, "Please help me! I can't breathe, and my heart is racing. I think I'm having a heart attack!" You help her sit down, then take her pulse, and find it to be 100 per minute, regular and strong; her respirations are 32 per minute. She tells you she has no pain, but asks the store manager to call an ambulance. As you're waiting for the ambulance, she tells you this has happened to her several times before, and that she has had an electrocardiogram, which showed normal cardiac function. Then she says, "But I *know* I'm having a heart attack! I'm so scared!"

a. How consistent are this woman's signs, symptoms, and risk factors with those of a cardiac problem?

IX. Practicing the Skill: Identifying Patterns

Definition. Interpreting what patterns of functioning are suggested by the data you've clustered together.

Why This Skill Promotes Critical Thinking

Identifying patterns is a major step toward identifying health problems. It helps you to form a beginning *picture* of the problems and to recognize gaps in data collection. Once you *recognize* gaps in data collection, you can decide how to focus assessment to gain that missing information.

Here's an example of identifying patterns of functioning and discovering missing pieces of information. Suppose you clustered together the following cues:

• No bowel movement in 3 days
• Abdominal fullness
• States he's been "constipated off and on for the past month"

You may recognize that these cues represent a pattern of *Altered Bowel Elimination*. Having recognized this pattern, you know to focus your assessment to gain more information to help you decide *exactly* what the problem with bowel elimination is. For example: You ask, "What does *off and on* mean?" The person responds, "I get so constipated I have to take lots of laxatives...then I get diarrhea." This added information is likely to make you suspect that the bowel elimination problem is being caused in part by laxative abuse. You can then explore his knowledge of using laxatives.

Guidelines: How to Accomplish This Skill

Identifying patterns requires knowledge of *usual function and risk factors* for abnormal function. For example, to recognize *abnormal* coping patterns, you need to know *normal* coping patterns; to recognize potential (risk) for abnormal coping patterns, you need to know the *risk factors* for abnormal coping patterns.

1. To identify patterns, analyze the cues you've clustered together, and decide whether they represent a pattern of normal, potentially abnormal, or abnormal function. The following explains how to know which of these are present:
   a. **Normal pattern of functioning:** You identified no signs and symptoms.
   b. **Potential (risk) for abnormal pattern of functioning:** You identified risk factors, but *no* signs and symptoms. For example, if your patient has little fiber intake, minimal exercise, and takes frequent laxatives, he has a potential (risk) for *Altered Bowel Elimination,* even if today he had a normal bowel movement.
   c. **Abnormal pattern of functioning:** You identified *signs and symptoms.* For example, your patient complains of constipation and hasn't had a bowel movement in 3 days.
2. Once you have a beginning idea of the patterns, ask yourself what *other* information might help you clarify your understanding of the pattern; then collect that information.

Practice Exercises: Skill IX

Consider the data listed for each letter a–e below. Then choose which one of the following patterns best describes the cluster of data, and explain why.

Potential (Risk) for Altered Bowel Elimination Pattern

Potential (Risk) for Altered Sexual-Reproductive Pattern

Normal Sleep-Rest Pattern

Altered Respiratory Function Pattern

Normal Coping Pattern

a. Bilateral rales; respirations increased to 34 per minute; coughing up thick, white mucus.
b. States, "I can cope with my illness, so long as I have help from my husband." Manages daily self-care; has husband cook all meals; passes the time by knitting blankets for the homeless.

c. Eats little roughage; drinks 2 glasses of water daily; spends most of her time in bed; normal bowel function.

d. Works nights; sleeps 4 hours in the morning and 3 hours just before going to work at night.

e. Has just been diagnosed with genital herpes; single; believes there's nothing wrong with single people having sex; worried about transmitting herpes to future sex partners and future children (during delivery).

X. Practicing the Skill: Identifying Missing Information

Definition. Recognizing gaps in data collection and filling in the gaps.

Why This Skill Promotes Critical Thinking

Recognizing gaps in information, and filling in those gaps, prevents you from making one of the most common critical thinking errors: making judgments based on incomplete information. It also helps you clarify your understanding of the situations at hand.

Guidelines: How to Accomplish This Skill

1. One of the best ways to identify missing information is to analyze your written information and ask, "What's missing here?" When you have all the information before you, your brain can more readily recognize what's missing than when going over the information mentally.

2. Other strategies for recognizing missing information include accomplishing all of the following critical thinking skills:
   a. Identifying assumptions (Skill I)
   b. Checking accuracy and reliability of data (Skill III)
   c. Clustering related cues (Skill VI)
   d. Recognizing inconsistencies (Skill VIII)
   e. Identifying patterns (Skill IX)

Practice Exercises: Skill X

Go back to the practice exercises for Skill IX. For each pattern represented by the information listed in a–e, decide what information might be missing that could add to your understanding of the pattern.

XI. Practicing the Skill: Identifying Actual and Potential (Risk) Problems/Supporting Conclusions with Evidence

Definition. Stating exactly what the existing and potential (risk) problems and their causes are; providing the evidence that led you to conclude that the problems are (or may become) present.

Why This Skill Promotes Critical Thinking

Clearly and specifically stating problems and their causes is the first step to problem-solving. When you're clear about the problems and their causes, you can better determine *specific actions* to monitor, prevent, resolve, or control them. For example, consider how much more you know about problem *b* below than *a:*

a. *Fluid Volume Deficit*
b. *Fluid Volume Deficit related to fever and decreased fluid intake*

Providing the supporting evidence that led you to conclude exactly what the problems are helps you and others evaluate thinking. For example, consider the two problem statements below. Which one helps you better evaluate whether the problem has been correctly identified?

a. *Fluid Volume Deficit*
b. *Fluid Volume Deficit related to decreased fluid intake as evidenced by statements of thirst and intake of only 500 ml in the last 24 hours.*

The importance of clearly stating the problems is emphasized when you consider what can happen if you misdiagnose health problems. If you make a diagnostic error (miss problems or name them incorrectly), it can cause can cause you to:

• Initiate actions that aggravate the problems or waste time.
• Omit essential actions required to solve the problems.
• Allow problems to go untreated.
• Influence others to believe the problems exist as described incorrectly.

Predicting potential (risk) problems greatly enhances critical thinking because it helps you identify ways of *preventing* the problems, and *manage* them if they do occur. The importance of predicting potential problems and complications is emphasized by the trend in health care to shift from a *diagnose and treat* philosophy to a *predict and manage* philosophy (you don't wait for problems to happen, you predict them and plan how to prevent and manage them).

Guidelines: How to Accomplish This Skill

As with most of these skills, your ability to identify and predict problems and complications depends on your knowledge and clinical expertise. If your knowledge and expertise are limited, you have an increased risk of making any one of the following common diagnostic errors:

• Overvaluing the probability of one diagnosis
• Not considering all the relevant data because of a narrow focus
• Failing to recognize personal biases or assumptions

- Making a diagnosis that's too general
- Overanalyzing and delaying taking action

Knowing that beginning nurses are at risk for the above mistakes helps them and more experienced nurses to *look* for these types of errors so that they can be corrected early.

The following guidelines are presented for identifying actual and potential (risk) problems:

To Identify Actual Problems (Nursing Diagnoses and Collaborative Problems)

1. Verify that your information is correct and complete.
2. Avoid drawing conclusions or identifying problems based on only one cue. The more cues you have to support your conclusions, the more likely it is that your conclusions are valid.
3. Cluster abnormal data (signs and symptoms): Cluster according to body systems to identify medical problems, and a nursing model to identify human response problems (nursing diagnoses).
4. Consider the signs and symptoms, and ask yourself what information you could have missed.
5. Create a list of suspected problems (nursing diagnoses and collaborative problems) that may be suggested by your patient's signs and symptoms. **If you're not sure where to start when trying to create a suspected problem list, REPORT SIGNS AND SYMPTOMS immediately to expedite problem identification and ensure patient safety.** Even if you don't understand the problems, reporting signs and symptoms is a valuable and important step in expediting treatment.
6. Compare your patient's signs and symptoms with the signs and symptoms or defining characteristics of the suspected problems.
7. Rule out problems that have signs and symptoms or defining characteristics that are *different* from your patient's signs and symptoms.
8. Name the problems by choosing the diagnoses that *most closely resemble* your patient's signs and symptoms.
9. Determine *underlying cause* (or related factors) of the problems:
   a. Always ask yourself whether it's possible that untreated (or inadequately treated) medical problems are causing the problems. If so, initiate a medical consultation immediately.
   b. Ask the person and significant others if they can identify factors that are contributing to the problems.
   c. Consider whether there are factors related to age, disease process, or life changes that could be contributing to the problems.
   d. Look up the diagnoses you've identified and check common related or causative factors; then assess your patient for the presence of any of these factors.

10. Using the mnemonic **PCE** (problem, cause, evidence), develop a problem statement that describes the:
    a. **P**roblem
    b. **C**ause (risk factors)
    c. **E**vidence that led you to conclude the problem exists
    d. Use *related to* to link the problem and its cause (e.g., *Pain Related to left rib fracture as evidenced by statements of extreme tenderness in the left rib cage area*).

To Predict Potential (Risk) Nursing Diagnoses

1. Cluster data that indicate risk factors (related factors) for problems. For example, you may cluster the following data: immobile, elderly, fragile skin.
2. Name the potential (risk) problem by stating the problem and the risk factors, using *related to* to link the problem and risk factors. For example:

Risk for Impaired Skin Integrity related to immobility and fragile skin

To Predict Potential Complications

Consider the medical problems present and determine common potential complications. For example, if your patient just had a myocardial infarction (MI), determine common potential complications of MI (congestive heart failure, arrhythmias, pericarditis, MI extension, and cardiac arrest). Problem statements for potential complications are usually described by using the letters *PC,* followed by a colon (Carpenito, 1993). For example:

PC: Hemorrhage   or   *PC: Increased Intracranial Pressure*

Practice Exercises: Skill XI

■ Scenario One

You've clustered together the following data: Mrs. Pue has just been told she has terminal cancer. She refuses to take her medications. She sleeps most of the time, and says she doesn't want to talk to anyone. Mrs. Pue states she's going to die so she'd rather not bother talking.

Based on the above information, choose between the following three likely nursing diagnoses, and write a problem statement using the PCE format:

Ineffective Individual Coping, Powerlessness, Hopelessness

■ Scenario Two

Elaine has just returned from the recovery room after having an appendectomy under general anesthesia. She's very groggy and extremely nauseated.

Based on the above information, predict the potential complications Elaine might experience.

■ Scenario Three

You've just admitted Nigel to the psychiatric unit. He is agitated, but won't talk to anyone. You check previous records, and note that he has a history of striking caregivers.

Develop a diagnostic statement that best describes this potential problem by stating the problem and its risk factors.

XII. Practicing the Skill: Setting Priorities

Definition. Differentiating between problems needing immediate attention and those requiring subsequent action; deciding what problems *must* be addressed in the plan of care.

Why This Skill Promotes Critical Thinking

Deciding what must be done *first* and what's *most important* helps you avoid an inefficient, possibly dangerous approach to problem-solving.

- If you miss treating immediate priorities, the problems may deteriorate to a situation that is more difficult to treat. It's also likely to prevent you from treating other problems adequately. For example, if someone is in pain, and you begin discharge teaching without resolving the pain (an immediate priority), there's likely to be very little learning.
- If you give equal attention to major and minor problems, you risk focusing inadequate attention on the *major problems that must be addressed* to meet the overall goals.

By identifying relationships between problems and treating the ones that are contributing to *other* problems first, you'll avoid "quick fixes" and develop a safe and effective plan that's more likely to achieve long-term beneficial results. A classic example of the risks "quick fixes" cause is when pain is treated without first determining and treating its cause.

Guidelines: How to Accomplish This Skill

As the definition above implies, setting priorities happens in two phases:

1. First, identify problems requiring immediate attention, and initiate treatment as indicated (see Display 3–7 on page 62).
2. Second, after initiating essential early treatment, determine what problems must be addressed on the plan of care in order to achieve the major goal of care:
   a. Determine an overall discharge goal (expected outcome). For example, "Client will return home able to manage health care independently." (How to determine expected outcomes is addressed in the next skill. To help you complete this sections, outcomes are provided for you.)
   b. Be sure you've identified underlying causes of the problems. *Causes* of problems should be assigned high priority: Preventing, resolving, or controlling the *causes* is essential to preventing, resolving, or controlling the *problems*.
   c. List the problems you've identified; then determine whether there are relationships between the problems (consider whether one problem is contributing to another). Place a high priority on problems that contribute to other problems.
   d. To help you set priorities among human response problems, use a method such as the one presented in Display 5–1.
   e. Assign a high priority to addressing the following problems on the plan of care: problems not covered by facility standard plans, protocols, or physician's orders; problems that might jeopardize achieving the major expected outcomes of the plan of care.

Practice Exercises: Skill XII

1. You've identified the discharge goal of "Will be discharged home by 7/28 able to perform his own colostomy care." Which *one* of the following problems should be addressed on the plan of care?
   a. *Anxiety related to inability to return to work for 6 weeks*
   b. *Knowledge Deficit: Colostomy care*
   c. *Risk for Impaired Skin Integrity Related to Colostomy*
2. Read the following scenarios, then answer the questions that follow them.

◼ Scenario One

Mr. Santos is a 64-year-old Guatemalan migrant worker who is admitted with a right calf thrombophlebitis. He is on bed rest, warm soaks, and anticoagulants. His knowledge of English is minimal. Today you're trying to teach him how to give himself anticoagulant injections. You're having real problems communicating, and you're thinking you should contact Social Services to try to get a transla-

| Display 5–1 | A Commonly Used Method of Setting Priorities for Human Responses (Maslow's Hierarchy of Human Needs) |

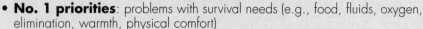

- **No. 1 priorities**: problems with survival needs (e.g., food, fluids, oxygen, elimination, warmth, physical comfort)
- **No. 2 priorities:** problems with safety and security needs (e.g., risks of injury or infection, threats to feeling secure)
- **No. 3 priorities:** problems with love and belonging (e.g., family problems, separation from loved ones)
- **No. 4 priorities:** problems with self-esteem needs (e.g., need for privacy, respect, independence, and positive self-image)
- **No. 5 priorities:** problems with self-actualization needs (e.g., need to grow and accomplish goals)

Summarized from Maslow, A. (1970). *Motivation in personality*. New York: Harper & Row.

tor to attend the teaching sessions. Mr. Santos is able to convey to you that his leg is still painful, and that he's also been getting pains in his chest.

Based on the above information, what's your most immediate priority?

■ Scenario Two

You're looking after Neil, a 16-year-old football player who had surgery for a ruptured spleen 14 hours earlier. He is alert, his vital signs are stable, and his abdominal dressing is clean and dry. He has some incisional discomfort, and hasn't been medicated for pain since surgery. He is also uncomfortable because he hasn't been able to void since surgery. He says, "I feel so lousy, I wish my mother could stay with me. She always makes me feel better." When you offer to call her, he replies, "No, she's dying of cancer. Would you call my aunt?"

1. You've identified the following needs/problems. Using Display 5–1 above as a guide, decide how you would prioritize the needs/problems below: Place a "1" (for first priority), "2" (second priority), or "3" (third priority) in the appropriate blank.
   a. ____ Wants his aunt to come in
   b. ____ Hasn't voided
   c. ____ Has incisional pain
2. Explain why you chose the order of priorities you listed above.
3. The discharge goal for Neil is "Will be discharged home by day 3 able to manage changing dry sterile dressings." Neil demonstrates dressing changes the day after surgery, and relates the importance of impeccable wound care. He is ambulatory and voiding well. Which *one* of the following *might* be addressed on the care plan, and why?
   a. *Risk for Infection related to incision*

b. *Anticipatory Grieving related to loss of his mother as evidenced by statements that mother has terminal cancer and he wishes she could be with him*
c. *Knowledge Deficit: Dressing changes*

XIII. Practicing the Skill: Determining Specific, Realistic, Client-Centered Goals (Expected Outcomes)

Definition. Deciding exactly what the client must be able to accomplish and by when he or she must be able to accomplish it.

Why This Skill Promotes Critical Thinking

"What's the goal of my thinking?" and "How much time do I have?" are two of the eight key questions you need to ask to determine your approach to critical thinking. Deciding exactly what the *client* is expected to accomplish helps you:

- Keep the focus on *client responses,* the most important barometer for measuring how well the plan is working (you measure progress by comparing client responses with expected outcomes).
- Determine *specific interventions* to achieve the outcomes.

Knowing by when outcomes are to be accomplished motivates the client and caregivers to initiate actions in a timely fashion. Being realistic about patient capabilities and what can be accomplished within the allotted time frame prevents frustration and helps you focus on *major priorities.*

Guidelines: How to Accomplish This Skill

To determine specific, realistic goals, first be sure you've clearly stated the problems: Goals are derived directly from the problem statements. If your problems are incorrectly identified or stated, your goals are likely to be incorrect.

Below are examples of nursing diagnoses and corresponding goals (outcomes). Notice how the statements on the *right* restate the problems on the *left* in a way that shows the problem is resolved or controlled.

Nursing Diagnosis	Appropriate Goal (Expected Outcome)
Ineffective airway clearance	Will demonstrate effective airway clearance as evidenced by demonstrating ability to clear lungs of secretions; and consistently demonstrating clear lungs

| **Knowledge deficit:** | Will explain and demonstrate key aspects of |
| **Newborn care** | newborn care as described in *Mothers' Newborn Care Pamphlet* |

| **Pain** | Will relate being pain-free or that pain level is managed to the point that it doesn't interfere with daily activities or sleep |

Only nursing diagnoses are listed above because outcomes for collaborative problems are usually addressed in standard facility plans (e.g., critical paths). However, the principles for goal setting provided below can be applied to *any* situation.

To identify specific, realistic, client-centered outcomes:

1. Establish an overall discharge goal (expected outcome).
   Example: By 1/6, will be discharged to home under care of his mother.
2. List priority problems that must be addressed on the plan of care (those that must be prevented, resolved, or controlled in order to be discharged by the date listed in the discharge goal).
3. Including the client and significant others, and any other involved caregivers as appropriate, develop a realistic, client-centered goal for each of the priority problems you identified:
   a. Restate the problem statements to reflect satisfactory improvement or resolution of the problems.
   b. Make sure the subject of your problem statement is the client or a part of the client. For example: "The *client* will ambulate independently" or "The *client's incision* will be free of signs of inflammation." If it's clear that the client is implied in the outcome statement, it's acceptable to omit the words *the client* (e.g., "Will ambulate independently").
4. Set specific dates for when you expect each outcome to be achieved. If the goal is on-going, no date is used: For example, "Will maintain normal bowel function."
5. If appropriate, use *as evidenced by* to describe exactly what you'll assess to decide if the outcome has been met.* For example: "The client will demonstrate knowledge of insulin management as evidenced by ability to: state how insulin works, perform glucose monitoring, adjust insulin dose according to blood sugar level, and use sterile injection technique."
6. Once the final outcomes are determined, share them with all the key players (patient, significant others, other caregivers) as appropriate to be sure that they're agreeable to those involved.
7. Make any changes as necessary, based on the above.

---

*Sometimes, *as evidenced by* becomes repetitive within the statement. In these cases, it can be omitted.

Practice Exercises: Skill XIII

For each problem below, determine a specific, client-centered outcome.

1. Risk For Impaired Skin Integrity related to age, obesity, and prolonged bed rest
2. Powerlessness related to quadriplegia as evidenced by statements of "I have no choices"
3. Activity Intolerance related to muscle weakness secondary to prolonged bed rest as evidenced by inability to walk the length of the hall without assistance

XIV. Practicing the Skill: Determining Specific Interventions

Definition. Identifying nursing actions to monitor, prevent, control, or resolve the problems and achieve the outcomes; predicting responses to nursing actions, weighing risks and benefits, and tailoring the actions to make them specific to the patient.

Why This Skill Promotes Critical Thinking

Identifying specific interventions designed to increase the likelihood of achieving the outcomes and decrease the likelihood of harm is essential to developing a safe and efficient plan. Imagining the risks of interventions helps you be proactive: You can "test" interventions mentally before putting the plan into action. Having predicted the risks, you can tailor the interventions to reduce them. Weighing the risks against the benefits helps you determine harmful interventions (you can decide whether your actions have a greater likelihood of causing harm than benefit).

Making your interventions specific increases the likelihood that the actions will be carried out in detail. It also provides a way to evaluate thinking. Consider the two interventions listed below. Notice how *b* demonstrates clear, detailed critical thinking, as compared with *a*.

a. Monitor breath sounds and help with coughing and deep breathing
b. Monitor breath sounds, splint front left lower ribs, and help with coughing and deep breathing every 4 hours during waking hours

Guidelines: How to Accomplish This Skill

1. Clearly state the problem.
   Example: Activity Intolerance *related to weakness and fatigue* after being on prolonged bedrest as evidenced by inability to ambulate to bathroom without assistance.
2. Develop a client-centered outcome. For example, "Will ambulate to the bathroom with a walker the length of hall by discharge."

3. Focus on the *related to* part (contributing or causative factors) of the problem statement. For example, the words in italics in No. 1 above.
4. Consider whether any causes require additional medical evaluation or treatment.
5. Ensure that any required medical evaluation or treatment is initiated.
6. Remembering the mnemonic M-PCR (**M**onitor, **P**revent, **C**ontrol, **R**esolve), determine *specific* actions that will:
    a. Monitor, prevent, resolve, or control the *cause* (risk factors) of the problem.
    b. Monitor, prevent, resolve, or control the *problem.*
7. If appropriate, ask the patient and significant others what they feel could be done to prevent, resolve, or control the problems.
8. Tailor the above interventions to increase the likelihood of achieving the expected outcome.
9. Predict responses to your interventions, and determine any risk of harm.
10. Fine tune the interventions to include ways of increasing the likelihood of beneficial responses and decreasing the risk of harm.
11. When you write the interventions, remember the words "see, do, teach, record": Consider what you'd *see* (assess), what you'd *do,* what you'd *teach,* and what you'd *record.* In the example in No. 1 above, your interventions might be like this:
    a. **See (assess)**. Assess ability to walk with walker in the room before allowing him to go out in the hall alone.
    b. **Do**. Have him walk the length of the hall three times a day.
    c. **Teach**. Reinforce that sticking to the plan will increase muscle strength and reduce fatigue.
    d. **Record**. Record pulse and blood pressure before and after walking at least once a day.

Practice Exercises: Skill XIV

1. Determine specific interventions for each of the following problems:
    a. Risk for Fluid Volume Deficit related to diarrhea and insufficient fluid intake.
    b. Anxiety related to insufficient knowledge of hospital procedures as evidenced by statements of becoming anxious when not warned and taught about procedures.
    c. Diarrhea related to medication side effects as evidenced by 6–8 loose stools daily.
    d. Chronic Pain related to arthritic joints as evidenced by statements of suffering from arthritic pain in knees and hands for the past 20 years.
    e. Impaired Communication related to slurred speech as evidenced by inability to enunciate words (can communicate in writing well).
2. Read the following scenario, then answer the questions that follow it.

■ Scenario

You're making a community health visit to the Supopoff's, Russian immigrants who are living in the suburbs in a church-sponsored home. The family has three children, aged 5, 7, and 10. The house they live in is adjacent to a tall grassy area, which is full of deer ticks. Mrs. Supopoff is upset because she keeps finding deer ticks on the children, and she knows about Lyme disease following deer tick bites. Even though she's told the children not to go into the grassy area, she suspects they disregard her instructions when playing. Mrs. Supopoff is considering punishing the children when she finds a tick on them, hoping this will make them be more careful.

You look up Lyme disease and learned that:

• Deer ticks are tiny (the size of a pin head).
• Lyme disease is *serious,* and the best treatment is *prevention* of tick bites.

You identify the following problem and goal:

• Problem: Risk For Infection related to tick bites
• Expected outcome: The children will have a decreased risk of getting tick bites and infection as evidenced by wearing insect repellant when outside, avoidance of tall grass areas, and monitoring themselves and each other for ticks.

1. Consider the risks and benefits of the following actions:
   a. What might happen if the children are punished when a tick was found on them?
   b. What might happen if you reward the children for finding ticks?
2. What interventions might safely motivate the children to participate in spotting ticks?
3. Write specific interventions to achieve the above expected outcome.

XV. Practicing the Skill: Evaluating and Correcting Our Thinking

Definition. Looking for flaws in our thinking, determining how well we've accomplished critical thinking skills, and making necessary corrections.

Why This Skill Promotes Critical Thinking

Critical thinking is active, purposeful thinking that strives for accuracy and reliability. As humans, our thinking is sometimes flawed. By *looking* for flaws, we can correct them early, increasing the likelihood of sound reasoning.

Guidelines: How to Accomplish This Skill

As discussed in previous skills, evaluating and correcting thinking is an *ongoing* process. Display 5–2 (next page) provides the types of questions you should be asking at various steps of the nursing process to evaluate and correct thinking.

There are no practice exercises for this skill, as opportunities for evaluating and correcting thinking have been provided throughout the other skills.

XVI. Practicing the Skill: Developing a Comprehensive Plan/Evaluating and Updating the Plan

Definition. Stating the priority problems, identifying specific client-centered outcomes, and determining interventions; determining client progress toward outcome achievement and making necessary changes in the plan of care.

Why This Skill Promotes Critical Thinking

Clearly documenting a comprehensive plan provides a basis for evaluation. When each step of the nursing process is recorded, you can more readily evaluate thinking and note discrepancies in the plan. For example, if someone isn't progressing toward outcome achievement, you can review the entire plan, looking for flaws and evaluating how decisions were made.

Evaluating progress toward outcome achievement helps you decide whether the plan requires changing, or whether it's even necessary to continue the plan.

Guidelines: How to Accomplish This Skill

Developing a comprehensive plan requires being able to accomplish the skills listed in this section, as you assess, diagnose, plan, implement, and evaluate care.

To evaluate progress toward outcome achievement, compare your patient's data with the established expected outcomes. For example, if the expected outcome states *will be free of signs of infection around wound incision,* assess the incision for signs of infection (e.g., redness, drainage, heat, tenderness).

Practice Exercises: Skill XVI

1. Consider each of the expected outcomes and corresponding patient data and decide whether the outcome has been achieved, partially achieved, or not achieved.

   a. **Expected outcome:** Will be ready for discharge by day 3 after surgery as evidenced by ability to relate how to manage wound

Display 5–2 **Examples of Questions Asked to Evaluate and Correct Thinking at Various Stages of the Nursing Process**

1. **Assessment**
   - What assumptions could we have missed?
   - How complete is data collection?
   - How sure are we of the accuracy and reliability of the data?
   - How well do we understand my patient's perceptions?
   - How sure are we of the conclusions I've drawn (inferences I've made)?

2. **Diagnosis**
   - How well does the evidence support that the problems we've identified are correct?
   - Have we missed any other problems that could be indicated by the evidence?
   - Did we make any value judgments?
   - Are we clear about the underlying causes?
   - How clearly and specifically are the problems stated?
   - Did we include human responses (nursing diagnoses) and collaborative problems?
   - Were client strengths and resources identified?

3. **Planning**
   - What immediate priorities could have been missed? Did we remember to include the patient and significant others in setting priorities?
   - Have we missed any problems that need to be addressed on the plan of care?
   - How well do the outcomes reflect an improvement or resolution of the identified problems?
   - Are the outcomes client-centered?
   - How specific and realistic are the outcomes? How realistic are the time frames set for goal achievement?
   - How specific are the interventions?
   - Did we remember to consider client preferences when developing the plan? Did we take advantage of client strengths and resources?

4. **Implementation**
   - Are the problems still the same?
   - Are we missing any new problems?
   - Are we keeping the focus on *client responses*?
   - Should we be doing anything differently? Are the interventions still appropriate?

5. **Evaluation**
   - How accurately and completely have we completed each of the previous steps?
   - What could we be doing differently?

packing. **Patient data:** Doesn't feel managing wound packing should be his concern, and feels he's incapable of doing so.

b. **Expected outcome:** Will drink at least 4 quarts of fluid as evidenced by keeping a written record of fluid intake. **Patient data:** Record indicates 5 quarts of fluid intake daily.

c. **Expected outcome:** The baby will be discharged home with parents able to perform CPR. **Parent's data:** Father demonstrates CPR well. Mother has trouble establishing airway.

2. Develop a comprehensive plan, identifying two priority diagnoses, for the following scenario. Include an overall discharge goal, client-centered outcomes for each diagnosis, and specific interventions.

■ Scenario

It's Monday. You admit Mrs. Kooney, who has just suffered anaphylactic shock after a bee sting. Mrs. Kooney is expected to be discharged by Wednesday. The doctor gives Mrs. Kooney an emergency epinephrine injection kit and tells her, "The nurse will teach you how to use it." Mrs. Kooney still has hives all over her body and says her itching feet are driving her crazy. You've found that placing her feet in cool water every so often really helps her discomfort. She is still slightly wheezy from the bee sting reaction.

When you ask her about using the injection kit, she replies "No way!" Her husband, who is retired, says, "I'll be glad to learn." It's decided that it's satisfactory to discharge Mrs. Kooney on June 29th, so long as her husband can demonstrate how to manage giving the epinephrine in an emergency.

RESPONSE KEY

The following are *example responses* for the end-of-chapter and practice exercises. If you have a question as to whether your responses are appropriate, check with your instructor.

End-of-Chapter Exercises

CHAPTER 1

3. (a) Paraphrasing any of the definitions beginning on page 9 or in Appendix A (page 146) is an appropriate response. (b) *Thinking* is basically *any mental activity*—it can be aimless and uncontrolled. Critical thinking is controlled, purposeful, and more likely to lead to obvious beneficial results. (c) Four reasons are listed on page 4. (d) Once you're aware of your thinking style—your usual approaches to gaining understanding and making decisions—and get in touch with your talents and blind spots, you can then find ways to improve. (e) Any of the characteristics listed in Display 1–2 on page 10 are appropriate. (f) Both critical thinking and problem-solving focus on finding effective solutions. Critical thinking requires a more *proactive* approach, focusing on: predicting, preventing, detecting, and managing problems; and on finding ways to improve things, even when they are satisfactory. For more clarification, see page 11. (g) See Display 1–3, page 12, Principles of Critical Thinking Similar to Principles of Science and the Scientific Method.

CHAPTER 2

1. Critical thinking is often enhanced by our ability to use resources and teach ourselves. If we know how to take advantage of our preferred learning styles, we'll learn more easily and efficiently.

2. Only *you* know what your preferred learning style is.
3. (a) See pages 20–27. (b) See pages 24–27. (c) See page 32. (d) If we can't communicate effectively, gain trust, and establish good interpersonal relationships, we have difficulty getting the facts we need to think critically. Critical thinking is often enhanced by teamwork; communication skills and interpersonal skills are essential to teamwork. (e) See page 30. (f) Any of the skills on pages 31–34 are good example responses. The skills can all be developed by *practicing*.

CHAPTER 3

1. You could irrigate a nasogastric tube if the facility permitted it, you've received permission from your instructor, you have the required knowledge and level of competence, the procedure is reasonable and prudent, and you're willing to assume accountability for how you performed the procedure and the patient response to the procedure.
2. See Display 3–6 (page 61).
3. In the hospital setting, realistic priorities are set by focusing only on problems that must be resolved in order for the person to be discharged from the hospital. In community and long-term care settings, more nursing diagnoses are addressed because there is more time, more family involvement, and nursing care focuses more on

optimum wellness, than simply curing disease.

4. (a) It's unlikely that the off-going nurse has really assessed the family's needs. It's highly unlikely that the family is doing fine. It appears as though the family has had limited involvement in the child's care. (b) You need to assess the family's needs and begin to include interventions that meet these needs in the nursing plan (e.g., allow the family to spend more time with the child).

5. (a) Critical thinking in nursing is similar to critical thinking in any situation in that it requires developing characteristics of critical thinkers, it's influenced by the factors addressed in Chapter 2, and it requires developing critical thinking skills. It's different in that the conclusions and decisions nurses make *affect people's lives:* There's less room for error, more risks, and a significant moral dimension to nursing's critical thinking. It also requires extensive knowledge of health problems (e.g., how they present and how they're prevented or managed). (b) **Critical thinking in nursing:** Entails purposeful, goal-directed thinking; aims to make judgments based on evidence (fact) rather than conjecture (guesswork); is based on principles of science and scientific method (e.g., maintaining a questioning attitude, following an organized approach to discovery, and making sure information is reliable); and requires strategies that maximize *human potential* (e.g., tapping on individual strengths), and compensate for problems caused by *human nature* (e.g., the powerful influence of personal perceptions, values, and beliefs). Some examples of when critical thinking is essential in nursing is when trying to: get a better understanding of something or someone; identify actual and potential problems; make decisions about an action plan; reduce risks of getting undesirable results;

increase the likelihood of achieving long-term beneficial results; find ways to improve (even when no problems exist). (c) **Goals of nursing:** To help people avoid illness and its complications; to help people gain an optimum level of independence and sense of well-being, regardless of health state (in cases of terminal illness, the goal of achieving a peaceful death is also appropriate). **Implications:** Because the conclusions and decisions we as nurses make *affect people's lives,* our thinking must be guided by sound reasoning—precise, disciplined thinking that promotes accuracy and depth of data collection, and seeks to clearly identify the issues at hand. Because we're committed to giving humanistic care, we must seek to help people within the context of *their* value systems, which may be different from our own; we must be keenly aware of the *moral* and *ethical dimensions* of our thinking. Because we're committed to achieving these goals in a cost-effective, timely fashion, we must constantly seek to improve both our personal ability to give nursing care *and* the overall efficiency of health care delivery. (d) Depending on your level of expertise, you may have addressed any one of the points listed in Table 3–1 on page 43. (e) Just as the problem-solving method provides a basis for precise, disciplined critical thinking in everyday situations, the nursing process provides the basis for critical thinking in nursing. (f) According to Tanner (1983), clinical judgment usually involves making a series of decisions that includes deciding: what to observe, what data suggest, what actions to take. del Bueno (1994) states that to practice safely, beginning nurses must be able to: identify essential data indicative of an acute change in health status; know why these actions are appropriate; differentiate between problems needing immediate attention and those requiring subsequent action; initiate independent and collaborative actions to correct or minimize risks to patients' health. (g) See Display 3–6, page 61. (h) Facility and national standards and guidelines are valuable tools to help you make care decisions. However, guidelines aren't meant to be followed *blindly*. An essential part of decision-making is using critical thinking to recognize when the situation at hand *differs* from the guide. (i) Any of the strategies listed beginning on pages 58–63 are correct.

CHAPTER 4

1. One of nursing's major goals is that of helping people be independent. It's our responsibility to teach them the information they need to know to be independent.
2. These terms are discussed on page 71.
3. See page 81 (strategies for memorizing effectively).
4. See page 83 (strategies for test-taking).
5. (a) Nurses are committed to giving humanistic care: We seek to help people within the context of their values and beliefs. When these values and beliefs are different from our own, we must decide when it's appropriate to express our opinion, and when we must withhold judgment. It's also not unusual for nurses to be involved in helping people make treatment decisions—decisions that have life-altering effects. Questions about who should have the right to make life-altering decisions are considered to be moral and ethical issues. (b) It's not unusual to be faced with moral and ethical issues that have no *right* answer: Rather, each answer has its own merits and risks with an equally uncertain outcome. (d) Any of the following: To think analytically about the situations they encounter and seek out research results that might improve nursing care; to raise questions about their practice that might prompt a researcher to formulate a question to guide a study; to help researchers collect data; to continue to acquire and share knowledge related to research. (f) You need to be able to recall facts to progress to higher levels of thinking, such as knowing how to apply and analyze information. Critical thinking, or reasoning our way through the learning process, helps us connect with our own unique way of making information ours. (g) You need to know yourself (your usual study and test-taking habits) to be able to identify ways of taking advantage of your strengths and compensating for your weaknesses. You need to know the content to be tested so that you can focus your attention on studying what's most important. Knowing the test format helps you know know how to prepare for the test (e.g., how much memorization you need to do), and helps you find ways of practicing for the test. Knowing test-taking skills helps you make the most of what you know and identify how to make educated guesses.

CHAPTER 5

Practice Exercises: Skill I

1. There's not enough evidence to support that the patient needs teaching. Many people are fully knowledgeable about their diet, but aren't able to stick to it.
2. You might waste your time teaching information the patient already knows. You might alienate the patient: Who likes to be taught things they already know? The patient gets the message that you don't understand the problem—that you jump to conclusions.
3. **Scenario One:** (a) She seems to have assumed that she can *create* a positive attitude for Jeff by talking about advances in diabetic care. (b) She needed to assess

Jeff's *human response* to learning he's a diabetic. Jeff may be well aware of advances in diabetic care, but still having trouble coming to terms with having to regulate his diet and take insulin for the rest of his life. She didn't *assess* before *acting.* (c) Jeff probably thinks Anita is a "know-it-all" because she didn't take the time to find out what his point of view on the situation was. It's a real turn-off when someone starts trying to change your attitude before they find out what your attitude *is.* **Scenario Two:** (a) She seems to have assumed the mother can read, and that the mother will let her know if she has questions. (b) If the mother can't read or is embarrassed to ask questions, the child may have inadequate care from his mother. If harm results from the nurse's failure to determine the mother's understanding, the nurse may be accused of negligence. **Scenario Three:** (a) That he would have the *desired* response to the drug without any adverse reactions. (b) It's likely that she was concerned that Mr. Frank wouldn't respond to the diuretic as expected—that he might experience an adverse reaction. (c) She probably thought the physician wouldn't like it if she challenged his judgment.

Practice Exercises: Skill II

1. Figure 3–2, the body systems approach to assessment (page 52), is probably the best method. Or you may choose the head-to-toe approach, clustering signs and symptoms of medical problems after you perform the assessment.
2. You should have chosen a nursing model approach. Nursing models can be found in Tables 3–2 and 3–3 (pages 47–48), and on pages 105–108 (unnumbered figure).
3. **Scenario One:** (a) Assess: the extent of Pearl's voluntary movement (can she wig-

gle her toes?); color of toes and skin around cast edges; whether Pearl feels numbness or tingling in her foot or leg; whether there is any edema of the leg or toes; the quality of the dorsalis pedis pulse; whether Pearl perceives a needle prick as being sharp; whether her toes are warm or cool. (b) Assessing each of the above helps you detect *early* signs of circulatory problems, nerve compression, or skin irritation: If you find one area that begins to exhibit abnormal assessment findings (e.g., edema), you might decide to increase the frequency and intensity of assessment of *other* areas (e.g, skin color). Specific relevance of each area of assessment follows:

Area of Assessment	Relevance
Movement, numbness, sensation	Monitors for nerve compression
Color, edema, pulses, warmth	Monitors circulation and skin condition

(c) Check circulation by assessing the dorsalis pedis pulse quality and capillary refill to toes; check for nerve compression by asking her to wiggle her toes. If these are satisfactory, you might choose to put a warm sock over the toes; encourage her to wiggle her toes frequently to increase the circulation, and continue to monitor her dorsalis pedis pulse, toe temperature, and toe sensation closely.

Scenario Two: (a) You'd look up digoxin in a reference, then assess as follows. **To assess for therapeutic effect:** Check to see if Mr. Wu's serum digoxin level is within therapeutic range (0.8–2 ng/ml). Determine status of cardiac symptoms, as compared with baseline (status of: apical/radial pulse rate and rhythm, lung sounds, urine output, edema, activity tolerance). **To assess for adverse reactions:** Check Mr. Wu for signs and symptoms of any of the adverse reactions listed in the drug reference. You'd also assess for contraindications and toxicity/overdose, as follows. **To assess for contraindications:** Check Mr. Wu for signs and symptoms of any of the contraindications listed in the drug reference. Most common contraindications for digoxin include: serum potassium levels < 3.5 mEq/L (increases the risk of toxicity); pulse rate less than physician-prescribed parameters; clinical signs of toxicity/overdose. **To assess for Toxicity/Overdose:** Check Mr. Wu for signs and symptoms of toxicity/overdose. Most common signs and symptoms of digoxin toxicity include: serum digoxin level > 2 ng/ml; atrioventricular block (PR interval > 0.24 sec); progressive bradycardia, nausea, vomiting, visual disturbances (blurring, snowflakes, yellow-green halos around images). (b) If no *therapeutic effect* is achieved by giving a drug, or if the person is experiencing *adverse reactions,* you need to question whether there needs to be a change in dosage, or whether the drug should be continued at all. If you identify contraindications to giving the drug, you need to withhold the drug. If you identify signs of toxicity/overdose, it's especially important to withhold the drug because you'd be *adding* to the toxicity/overdose problem.

Scenario Three: (a) **Vital signs:** Take temperature, pulse, respirations, and blood pressure. **Eye opening:** Call Gerome's name, tell him to open his eyes; if no response, pinch him. **Best motor response:** Ask him to move each extremity; use a pin prick or pinch him and see if he can tell you where he feels it; if no response, pinch him and note whether he flexes his extremity to withdraw from pain, flexes in spasm, or extends his extremity. **Best verbal response:** Ask him what his name is, where he is, and what

day it is. **Pupillary reaction:** Determine size of each pupil in millimeters before flashing a light into it; then flash a light into *each* pupil and observe whether it constricts briskly. **Purposeful limb movement:** Check each extremity by asking Gerome to move it, observing for muscle contraction (attempts to move), ability to lift extremity, and ability to lift extremity even though you try to hold it down. **Limb sensation:** Prick each limb with a sterile needle and ask Gerome what he feels (this may be unnecessary for Gerome, since he has a head injury, rather than a spinal cord injury). **Seizure activity:** Observe for muscle twitching. **Gag reflex:** Place a clean tongue blade in the back of Gerome's throat and see if it triggers gagging. (b) By assessing all of these parameters, signs and symptoms of increased intracranial pressure can be detected early. Signs and symptoms of increased intracranial pressure are: decreasing level of consciousness, increased restlessness, irritability and confusion, increased headache, nausea and vomiting, increasing speech problems, pupillary changes (dilated and nonreactive or constricted and nonreactive pupils), cranial nerve dysfunction, increasing muscle weakness, flaccidity, or coordination problems; seizures; decerebrate posturing (muscles stiff and extended, head retracted) and decorticate posturing (muscles rigidly still, with arms flexed, fists clenched, and legs extended)—these are both *late* signs of increased intracranial pressure. (c) Monitor *other* parameters of neurologic assessment closely for *other* signs of increased intracranial pressure. If there are no *other* changes, and you can indeed arouse Gerome, you don't need to be immediately concerned; however, you should increase the frequency of assessment of all parameters until you're comfortable that the increased somnolence is merely a sign of the combined effects of fatigue and *existing* brain swelling (rather than increasing brain swelling). If you have ANY QUESTIONS about how to proceed, report the increased somnolence to your supervisor. (d) Check other neurologic parameters closely and report and record findings immediately; increase the frequency of assessment. (e) If the baseline pulse was rapid, this may be a normal finding. However, you should closely assess all the other assessment parameters to check for other reportable signs and symptoms. If the pulse is dropping to 60 beats per minute, closely monitor all the other assessment parameters and report the findings *immediately* (may be a sign of life-threatening increase in intracranial pressure).

Practice Exercises: Skill III

1. Talk with the patient and explore her feelings and concerns.
2. Ask him to take it again now (quietly observe his technique). If he is proficient at performing a check for blood glucose, it's likely his previous result was correct. If the second reading is significantly different from the previous reading, consider whether there is a relationship between the change in blood sugar reading and recent food intake or peak insulin levels. I would consider the blood sugar reading the patient took with you observing as being most valid.
3. Take it in the right arm.
4. Explore with the patient why he thinks he got his foot ulcers. Ask him to tell you what he does to avoid getting foot ulcers.

Practice Exercises: Skill IV

1. (a) If you assumed this was an oral temperature, you should have "S" here. You may have placed question mark here, which is actually a more correct response. You need to ask: *How was this temperature taken (orally, rectally, tympanic?)* (b) If you assumed the patient never has rales, you should have an "S" here. You may have placed question mark here, which is actually a more correct response. You need to ask questions like: *What do the patient's lungs sound like when he's in his usual state of health? What is the respiratory rate? How far up the back can you hear the rales? Are there just a few rales or copious rales? When the patient coughs, do the rales clear?* (c) You may have put an "S" here, but *you really need to ask if this is a normal pattern for the person and why the person only sleeps 3 hours at a time (e.g., it's not unusual for mothers of newborns to sleep only 3 hours at a time because of feeding schedules).* (d) S. (e) "O" or question mark. This is usually a normal finding, but you may have placed a question mark because you wanted to know such things as *whether there's any drainage, whether the area is hot to touch, and whether the patient is afebrile.* (f) O. This is normal for a 2-year-old. (g) S. (h) You may have placed an "S" here, but a better response is a question mark. You need to ask: *What are the bathing practices of a person of this culture?* (i) S. This is likely to be a normal finding, since the dialysis takes over the work of the kidney. (j) S or question mark. The pulse is somewhat slow, but might be normal for someone who is young and athletic or older and on cardiac medication. You may have wanted to ask: *What is this person's normal pulse?* or *Is the person taking any cardiac medications that slow the heart rate?*
2. The italicized words above provide examples of what else you might have wanted to know.

Practice Exercises: Skill V

1. (a) I suspect this information indicates infection of some sort. (b) I suspect this information indicates financial problems, *or*.... (c) I suspect this information indicates that the patient has trouble sticking to his diet. (d) I suspect this information indicates that the child wants to be sure his mother approves of his answer, or perhaps he is afraid. (e) I suspect this information indicates there is some medical reason for the grandmother's confusion.

Practice Exercises: Skill VI

Scenario One: (a) Stung by a bee on the ear an hour ago; ear has no stinger, is red and swollen; no rash or wheezing, normal pulse and respirations. (b) Afraid he might die; wants to have a popsicle and watch TV. (c) Didn't make sure she had parents' phone number down (investigate whether this was lack of knowledge or oversight); doesn't know first aid for a bee sting. **Scenario Two:** (a) 41 years old; acute abdominal pain; vomiting for 2 days, and unable to keep any food down; abdomen distended; no bowel sounds; scheduled to go to the operating room at 2 P.M.; pain suddenly getting worse; vital signs unchanged, except pulse is increased by approximately 30 beats/min. (b) 41-year-old businessman; hates everything about hospitals; scheduled to go to the operating room at 2 P.M.; worried because his brother died in the hospital after a car accident; suddenly experiencing *severe* pain.

Practice Exercises: Skill VII

Scenario One: (a) May be relevant because buspirone hydrochloride can cause confusion in the elderly. (b) May be relevant because it may be sign of infection, which can cause confusion in the elderly. (c) May be relevant

because it's indicative of previous cardiovascular disease, which is a risk factor for cerebrovascular accident (stroke), which may be the cause of the confusion. (d) May be relevant because dehydration in the elderly can cause electrolyte imbalance and confusion. (e) Not relevant (not abnormal). (f) Not relevant (not abnormal). **Scenario Two:** (a) Probably relevant. It takes time to adjust to a diabetic regimen. (b) Not relevant (not abnormal). (c) May be relevant (may feel constipation is caused by new diet). (d) May be relevant because she has to prepare meals for others, increasing temptation. (e) Very probably relevant. Someone who likes to cook usually takes joy in eating a variety of foods. (f) Relevant. She needs to eat even less than she will when her weight is within normal limits. (g) Not relevant (has nothing to do with sticking to a diabetic diet).

Practice Exercises: Skill VIII

Scenario One: (a) It doesn't make sense that she has only just started coming to prenatal clinic, but has been going to birthing classes. If she hasn't had prenatal care until now, you wonder whether she's really happy about the baby coming or realizes the importance of prenatal visits. You may also wonder why her mother, rather than her boyfriend, came to the clinic visit. (b) Check her records to see if there's any mention of receiving prenatal care somewhere else for the earlier part of her pregnancy; ask her where she's been going to birthing classes; ask how her boyfriend and mother feel about the baby coming. **Scenario Two:** (a) Her age is inconsistent with risk factors for a myocardial infarction (MI). The *big picture* here—her age, absence of pain, and previously normal electrocardiogram—is inconsistent with the big picture of an MI. *Occasionally* individuals don't have pain when they have an MI, but usually there are other risk factors and signs and symptoms present. Her signs and symptoms are more consistent with those of a panic attack.

Practice Exercises: Skill IX

(a) Pattern of Altered Respiratory Function. Signs and symptoms of respiratory function problems are present. (b) Normal Coping Pattern. There are no signs or symptoms of abnormal coping pattern. (c) Pattern of Potential (Risk) for Altered Bowel Elimination. There are risk factors for constipation present, but no signs and symptoms. (d) Normal Sleep-Rest Pattern. Considering the person works nights, there are no signs and symptoms of an abnormal sleep-rest pattern. (e) Potential (Risk) for Altered Sexual-Reproductive Pattern. There are risk factors for Altered Sexual-Reproductive Pattern.

Practice Exercises: Skill X

(a) What are the person's *other* vital signs (pulse, blood pressure, temperature)? Is there a history of smoking? Is the person smoking now? How long has this pattern persisted? What does the person feel is contributing to this pattern? How does the person tolerate activity? (b) How does the husband feel about helping the patient? (c) Who is the major caregiver in this case? What factors are contributing to the lack of roughage in diet and inadequate fluid intake? What's the patient's (or caregiver's) knowledge of how to prevent altered bowel elimination? Why does the patient spend most of his time in bed? How motivated is the patient to do the things necessary to prevent altered bowel elimination? (d) Does the person feel he's getting adequate rest? Does the patient take sleeping aids? If so, what are they? (e) What are the woman's feelings about hav-ing herpes? What's the woman's knowledge about herpes transmission? How does she feel about telling prospective partners about the herpes? How does the patient plan to prevent herpes transmission?

Practice Exercises: Skill XI

Scenario One: Hopelessness related to new diagnosis of terminal cancer as evidenced by withdrawn behavior (sleeps most of the time, doesn't want to talk to anyone). Powerlessness is also an acceptable response. There is a fine line between these two diagnoses. **Scenario Two:** Potential complications: hemorrhage, shock, vomiting with aspiration, pneumonia, infection, paralytic ileus. **Scenario Three:** Potential for (or Risk for) Violence related to agitation and previous history of striking caregivers when angry.

Practice Exercises: Skill XII

1. b. *a* is more likely to be dealt with informally or at home. *c* will be covered by the diagnoses listed in *b*.
   Scenario One: Reporting the chest pain should be your immediate priority. Myocardial infarction and pulmonary embolus, both serious problems, are potential complications of thrombophlebitis.
   Scenario Two:
1. (a) 3. (b) 2 or 3 is acceptable. (c) 2 or 3 is acceptable.
2. (a) According to the display, this is a No. 3 priority. (b) According to the display, this is a No. 1 priority. (c) According to the display, this is a No. 1 priority.
3. b. Unlike *a*, this isn't a routine diagnosis for someone who has an incision; *a* is also likely to be covered in standard policies. *c* is inappropriate because Neil knows how to change his dressing.

Practice Exercises: Skill XIII

1. Client will maintain intact skin, free of signs of redness or irritation. **2.** Client will express feelings about powerlessness and relate increased sense of power over his situation as evidenced by statements that he is allowed to make as many choices about his own care as possible. **3.** Will demonstrate increased activity tolerance as evidenced by ability to walk the length of the hall and back by 6/6.

Practice Exercises: Skill XIV

1. (a) Record intake, output, and number of stools every 8 hours. Increase clear liquid intake to 1 1/2 quarts during day shift (1 quart on evening shift, and 1/2 quart on night shift). Give anti-diarrheal as ordered prn. Stress to the patient the importance of maintaining adequate fluid intake. Record intake and output every 8 hours. (b) Ask the patient to describe anxiety level. Encourage her to express feelings and concerns. Explain all procedures. (c) Monitor number of stools in 24 hours. Report diarrhea to physician and ask whether drug dosage or drug can be changed. Give anti-diarrheal prn as ordered and record response. (d) Monitor pain level using a 0–10 scale (0 = no pain; 10 = severe pain). Give analgesic before doing range of motion activities. Encourage active range of motion exercises during periods of optimum comfort and during warm baths. Record pain level and ability to move joints. (e) Monitor ability to enunciate words. Ensure the slurred speech has been evaluated by a physician. Consider whether a speech pathologist should be consulted. Be patient and give her enough time to speak.

Allow her to write messages when she is tired or frustrated.

1. (a) It's quite likely the children won't report finding ticks, increasing the likelihood that the mother won't know when the children may have been bitten. It also increases the likelihood that the ticks won't be properly disposed of. I doubt that there will be benefits from using this approach (punishment). (b) It's possible that they may go *looking* for ticks, increasing the likelihood of being bitten. It's also possible that this approach might work, but the risks outweighs the benefits. **2.** Determine children's understanding of the severity of the consequences of tick bites and the importance of finding ways to avoid them. Initiate teaching as indicated. Explain to the children that they can best help by asking for insect repellant to be applied before going outside, reporting ticks found on themselves and on each other, and avoiding tall grass areas. Start a rule that the children can't go outside without first applying insect repellant. Have the mother praise good behavior (e.g., asking for insect repellant) verbally, rather than offer rewards. Instruct the mother not to offer rewards for finding ticks.

Practice Exercises: Skill XVI

1. (a) Not achieved. (b) Achieved. (c) Partially achieved, focus teaching toward mother's needs.
2. A comprehensive plan that lists two priority problems for the scenario follows:
Discharge Outcome: Will be discharged home with husband able to demonstrate administration of epinephrine by 6/29.
Nursing Diagnosis No. 1: Knowledge Deficit (Husband): Epinephrine administration.

Expected Outcome: Mrs. Kooney's husband will relate knowledge of action and side effects of epinephrine, when to administer epinephrine and demonstrate subcutaneous injection technique.

Interventions: Provide husband with literature about epinephrine administration. Assess husband's knowledge of epinephrine action, side effects, and administration. Also determine preferred learning style. Reinforce what he already knows; teach gaps in knowledge using the husband's preferred learning style. Record husband's progress toward expected outcome after each teaching session.

Nursing Diagnosis No. 2: Altered comfort (itching feet) related to hives as evidenced by hives over feet.

Expected Outcome: Patient will experience decreased itching as evidenced by statements of increased comfort.

Interventions: Assist patient to place feet in cool water prn. Medicate as ordered prn for itching.

Note: You may have chosen another diagnosis, such as *Ineffective Coping,* for Mrs. Kooney, in hopes that you can help her cope with the possibility of learning how to give her own injections.

Definitions of Critical Thinking

- A composite of skill development, knowledge of the subject, and attitude of the practitioner (Watson and Glaser, 1964).*
- Reasonable reflective thinking that's focused on what to believe or do (Ennis, 1987; Kintgen-Andrews, 1991)
- Purposeful and goal-directed thinking (Halpern, 1984)
- The art of thinking about your thinking while you are thinking in order to make your thinking better; more clear, more accurate, or more defensible (Paul, 1992)†

- An investigation whose purpose is to explore a situation, phenomenon, question, or problem to arrive at a hypothesis or conclusion about it that integrates all available information that can therefore be convincingly justified (Kurfiss, 1988)
- The skill and propensity to engage in an activity with reflective skepticism (McPeck, 1981)

---

* Edward Glaser is one of the earliest pioneers in critical thinking, publishing *An Experiment in the Development of Critical Thinking* in 1941. Together with Watson, he also developed the *Critical Thinking Appraisal Manual* (1964), the predominant instrument used for research on critical thinking in nursing prior to 1994. Many now believe that this tool does *not* measure critical thinking in nursing.

† Paul is considered to be one of the foremost authorities on critical thinking.

What's Your Preferred Learning Style?

Overall Categories: Doer (kinesthetic), visual learner (observer, reader), auditory learner (listener)

Specific Categories: Logical learner, linguistic learner, spatial learner, musical learner

Almost everyone is a combination of two or more of these styles.

Doers (Kinesthetic Learners): Learn best by doing, moving, experiencing, or experimenting. For example, they'd rather play with a syringe and inject a dummy before reading the procedure.

Strategies to Take Advantage of Your "Doing" Style

1. Ask if you can start by *doing* (e.g., fiddling with equipment before reading about how to use it). Observing, reading, and listening will be more meaningful after you *do*.
2. Be sure you know the risks of doing first, and find ways to minimize them (e.g., If you're playing on the computer, make sure you can't inadvertently erase a file).
3. When taking notes, use arrows to show relationships.
4. Pace up and down while reciting information to yourself.
5. Make tapes with the information you're trying to learn and play them while exercising (e.g., riding a bike), or read while riding a stationary bike.
6. Write key words in the air; use your fingers to help you remember (bend the forefinger as you memorize a concept,

then the bend the next for the next concept, and so on).
7. Change positions frequently while studying; take frequent short breaks involving activity. This doesn't mean chatting with friends—it's too easy to get side-tracked.
8. Study in a rocking chair.
9. Study with background music.
10. Ask if you can do assignments in an active way (e.g., create a poster, be part of a discussion group).

Visual Learners: Learn best by watching first. For example, they'd rather *watch* someone give an injection before reading the procedure.

Strategies to Take Advantage of Your "Visual" Style

1. Ask to be included in observational experiences.
2. Sit in the front of the room, so you stay focused on the teacher, not what's going on around you.
3. Take lots of notes, and use a highlighter. Recopy your notes when you're studying.
4. In skills labs, don't go first. Rather, watch your classmates, and take a later turn.
5. Read procedures through, focusing on illustrations.
6. Visualize procedures *in your mind's eye*, rather than trying to follow individual steps.
7. Write things down (e.g., things to be done, directions).
8. When learning new terms or concepts, or trying to remember something, write them on "sticky notes" and put them

147

where you'll see them frequently (the bathroom mirror, the computer).

9. Preview chapters by scanning headings and illustrations.

Auditory Learners: Learn best by hearing.

Strategies to Take Advantage of Your "Auditory" Style

1. Read by subvocalizing (mouth the words and almost whisper) and concentrate on hearing the words. This is especially important when reading test questions.
2. Just *listen* in class, focusing on hearing what the teacher *says* without taking notes; then make a copy of someone else's notes.
   - Tape classes, and listen to the tapes two or three times before exams.
   - Ask if you can give an oral report or hand in an audio tape for extra credit.
   - Memorize by making up songs or rhymes.
   - Study with a friend, so you verbalize the information.
   - Tape yourself as you read key information out loud, then listen to the tapes.

Logical Learners: Like to have things organized and consistent.

Strategies to Take Advantage of Your "Logical" Style

1. Recognize that organization and logical flow of content may be unique to each person: The way you might organize information might not be how someone *else* might organize it, even though both ways are useful.
2. When reading texts, jot down headings on separate pieces of paper, then write notes under the appropriate heading as you encounter information that belongs there.

This way, the chapter will be organized how *you* want it to be.

3. Organize and reorganize your notes.
4. Study in an orderly environment.
5. Put your notes on computer, so that they can readily be reorganized; print out each organization and compare them.

Linguistic Learners: Love words and new vocabulary.

Strategies to Take Advantage of Your "Linguistic" Style

1. When writing papers, come back to the paper and see what words you can get rid of (you probably have too many).
2. Take notes as you read, writing key points down; then study your notes, rather than the book, or you may have trouble focusing on key points.

Spatial Learners: Like less words and more boxes and diagrams.

Strategies to Take Advantage of Your "Spatial" Style

1. Put boxes around key information.
2. Diagram concepts you're trying to remember.
3. Recopy notes, using only key words.

Musical Learners: Like to hum, sing, play instruments.

Strategies to Take Advantage of Your "Musical" Style

1. Study while listening to favorite music. Remember what music you were listening to when studying specific content.
2. Go over information you want to remember in your head while playing an instrument.
3. Have someone read you the information while you're playing an instrument.

Mollan-Masters, R. (1992). *You are smarter than you think*. Ashland, OR: Reality Productions.

Robinson, A. (1993). *What smart students know: Maximum grades, optimum learning, minimum time*. New York: Crown Trade Paperbacks.

Improving Writing Through Critical Thinking

Once I asked someone, "Do you know how to get rid of writer's block?" He replied, "Yeah. You sit in front of the computer and stare at the blank screen until beads of sweat form on your forehead and you sweat it out."

We all know writing isn't easy—it takes patience and perseverance. But it can be *easier* if we know some simple writing strategies. As schools focus more on evaluating critical thinking, you can expect to be asked to do more writing assignments, and take more short-answer and essay tests (as opposed to multiple choice tests) than ever before. This is because there are really only two ways for faculty to know *how* you think: They can ask you to explain your thoughts orally or in writing. Until oral tests and assignments become convenient, asking you to write seems to be the best answer.

With a little work, you can learn to write better with less difficulty. As you improve your writing, you'll become more in touch with how to use your brain to think things through—you'll improve your grades and your ability to think critically.

The following strategies are provided to help you improve your writing skills through critical thinking. These strategies are more effective and reliable than "sweating it out."

General Strategies

1. **Get over "writing anxiety."** Lots of us have had bad experiences as youngsters and have developed attitudes like "I'm hopeless" or "Let's do something else." Get a tutor or take a course and *practice*. If you *believe* you're hopeless, you can be sure that you'll be right. Like any skill, good writing takes work and gets easier with practice. If you like to write letters or tell stories, you're probably a natural writer.

2. **Learn to type and use a word processor or computer.** Your mind works faster than your hand can write. A word processor allows your thoughts to flow freely, reduces frustration, and helps you revise quickly, making writing easier and more rewarding. There are lots of easy-to-learn writing programs available. If you're still writing by hand, it's as if you're walking to your destinations instead of taking the car.

3. **Use headings, even when asked to provide short answers.** For example, if you're asked to address two major goals of nursing, make each goal a heading. Headings help *you* to stay on track and help *readers* know what's coming up. Imagine this appendix without headings!

4. **When you find yourself struggling** to write long sentences or paragraphs, consider whether bullets or numbered points could express the information more easily:
   • See how easy it is to read these short points?
   • Our brains do better with short phrases or sentences than long ones.
   • Bulleted points are actually also easier to write.

5. **Use examples and analogies.** These help you make your point and show why your information is relevant.

6. **Develop your own style.** Don't be afraid

to let your personality come through, rather than sticking to strict rules of formality.

Strategies for Formal Papers

1. **Give yourself enough time** to complete the following steps.
   - **Plan:** Determine your theme and set a schedule.
   - **Write:** Write your paper according to the plan (you may, however, change the plan somewhat as you write if necessary; the point is to start with some sort of plan).
   - **Revise:** Evaluate and improve.
   - **Edit:** Proofread and correct.
2. **Before starting the assignment, carefully review your instructor's requirements and make a checklist of what seems to be most important to do.** Keep the checklist in a place where you readily see it (e.g., at the front of your notebook or beginning of your computer file for the paper). Refer to the checklist frequently to make sure you're focusing your paper in such a way that it meets the most important criteria being graded.

   The following is an example checklist:

   ### Checklist

   - 25% of grade is on description of nursing theory.
   - 50% of grade is on analysis and application of nursing theory.
   - 25% of grade is on format (grammar, spelling, bibliography).
   - Make sure to focus on how the theory can be applied *today*.
   - Use lots of examples.
3. **Start by discovering your thoughts and ideas** without being concerned about grammar or spelling.
   - List key ideas and questions that come to mind. Then review your ideas and ask yourself, "What questions or thoughts do these ideas raise?" Write these questions and thoughts down too.
   - Share your thoughts, feelings, and perceptions with friends. Ask them what questions or thoughts are raised for *them*.
   - If you express yourself well orally, put your thoughts on a tape recorder, then take notes on new ideas as you listen to yourself.
   - Keep a running list of your own ideas and ideas you've found interesting when reading (be sure to cite your references in your notes, or you might forget where the information came from and be accused of plagiarism).
   - Do your bibliography as you go along. When you encounter an interesting reference, immediately write down the full citation.
4. **Develop *one* central idea, issue, or theme** that you can explain to someone in two or three sentences.
5. **Make an outline, or simply list headings** of things you want to cover. Once you've listed your headings, number them in order of importance, then decide a logical flow of headings.
6. **Write first draft in as concentrated a time as possible,** with as few interruptions as possible. Be realistic—this doesn't mean pulling an "all-nighter."
7. **As you write, visualize your reader** (usually your instructor) in your mind's eye: Predict what he or she will want to know, and provide the information. If you don't want to visualize your instructor, visualize someone else you know who is inquisitive.
8. **Remember the "Three T's."**
   - **T**ell them what you're going to tell them (introduction).

- **T**ell them (body).
- **T**ell them what you told them (summary).

9. **Once you've written first draft, revise and improve,** preferably a few days later, to give yourself a "fresh eye." **Revising is as important as writing a first draft:** It's when you apply critical thinking to your own work and challenge yourself to write (and think) more clearly. Revising entails asking yourself questions like:

    - How well is the central idea of the paper addressed *early* in the paper? Somewhere early in the paper you should have something like, "The purpose of this paper is . . ." or "This paper addresses . . . ." (use these exact words). It won't be unusual to find a strong statement of this sort buried in the middle of your first draft (probably because your mind was "on a roll" at that point) or at the end, when you were making your final statements. Move these statements to the introduction.
    - How does my paper compare with my initial checklist of key points (see No. 2 above)?
    - How logical is the flow of my headings?
    - How well do my paragraphs stick to the headings?
    - How persuasively have I made my points or explained why I've come to the conclusions I've presented? (For example, writing, "I've struggled with these issues and have decided . . . because . . . .")
    - How clearly does my summary describe what the paper addressed?

10. **Edit your paper,** checking for grammar and spelling problems.
    - Have someone else proofread your paper. You won't be able to proofread it well because you've looked at it too often and too long.
    - If you can't get someone else to proofread, READ YOUR PAPER OUT LOUD, or you'll miss important corrections. When you read silently, your brain "edits" without your realizing it. When you read your paper *out loud,* you'll *hear* your mistakes.
    - Proofread more than once—once for general errors, then a second time looking for the types of errors you tend to make. (For example, I tend to typo "your" instead of "you're.")
    - Play GOOMP (Get Out Of My Paper): Go through the paper finding words, phrases, or sentences you can get rid of. When we write, we tend to add unnecessary words that can make it difficult for others to understand what's important. Compare the clarity of *a* and *b* below. I played GOOMP with *a* to get *b*.
      a. Altogether too many students feel that writing should be taught only to those people who want to go into journalism once they have finished school. What these students don't realize is that their efforts in practicing writing can greatly enhance their general ability to think critically.
      b. Many students feel that writing should be taught only to those who want to go into journalism. What these students don't realize is that practicing writing can enhance critical thinking.
    - Play ICM (I Caught Me): Check yourself for repetition. We tend to use the same words over and over, making them lose their impact. Sometimes, we even write two sentences back to back that essentially say the same thing.

Compare the clarity of *a* and *b* below. I played ICM with *a* to get *b*.

a. When thinking about how to write, think about what's most important. If you focus you're thinking about what's most important, you'll improve your thinking and your grades.

b. When writing, stay focused on what's most important. You'll clarify your thoughts and improve your grades.

In *a* above, I recognized there were too many "think's" and "thinking's," and found ways of getting rid of them.

11. **First impressions matter: Make it look good.** Check your margins and spacing. If you're hand-writing your paper, you might want to write it with a pencil so you can erase—then hand in a photocopy so that it's cleaner and looks as though it was written in ink.

Strategies for Getting Over Writer's Block

1. **Just get started,** letting your ideas flow onto the paper (or into the computer in whatever order they come to you). Sometimes, writing is like exercising. You need a warm-up period.

2. **Break the paper down into small tasks.** For example, if you can't seem to get started on the introduction, go on to address some of your other headings. It's not unusual to write the best introduction once you've finished your paper. Doing easier headings first reduces your anxiety, helps you see progress, and gets your brain in "writing gear."

3. **"Talk through" your paper.** Call a friend and say, "I'm stuck on a point for my paper. Can you listen so I can explain it to you?" Write down key points as you explain them.

Examples of: Critical Path, Data Base Assessment Tool, Neurological Focus Assessment Tool, Neurovascular Focus Assessment Tool

APPENDIX D—FRACTURED HIP CLINICAL PATHWAY

CARE NEED	DAY 4 - POD 2	Done	Var	DAY 5 - POD 3	Done	Var	DAY 6 - POD 4	Done	Var	DAY 7 - POD 5	Done	Var
ASSESSMENT	DATE: Neurovasc check q shift & prn / *Sequential Compression Device / *TED stockings-off 1 hr q shift / Mentation clear; 02 prn; IS/CDB prn; breath sounds clear / *02 sat. if new onset confusion < 90-notify MD ___ / T < 38C; Skin check q shift / *Change dressing ___ / *DC wound drain			DATE: Neurovasc check q shift & prn / *Sequential Compression Device / *TED stockings-off 1 hr q shift / Mentation clear / Breath sounds clear / T < 38 / Dressing dry and intact/change prn / Skin Intact			DATE: Neurovascular check q shift & prn / *Sequential Compression Device / *TED stockings-off 1 hr q shift / Mentation clear / Breath sounds clear / T < 38 / Dressing dry and intact/change prn / Skin Intact			DATE: Neurovascular check q shift & prn / *TED stockings-off 1 hr q shift / Mentation clear / T < 38C / Dressing dry and intact/change prn / Skin Intact		
PAIN	PO Meds / Pharm consult if new confusion			PO Meds			PO Meds			PO Meds		
MOBILITY ENDO NSG:	Turn q 2-3 hrs while in bed with wedge			Recliner × 1 (3-11) / Wedge @ NOC			Wedge prn/pillows / Increase ambulation			Increase ambulation		
PT:	Exercises per protocol / Ambulate to chair / OT consult, if necessary / Weight Bearing Status: ___ P.T.			Exercises per protocol / Increase ambulation / Start home exercise program ___ P.T.			Exercises continued / Increase ambulation / Bathroom transfer ___ P.T.			Exercises continued / Increase ambulation / Stairs/crutches, prn / Car transfer @ D/C ___ P.T.		
ORIF NSG:	Transfer bed to chair w/2 assists			Ambulate 3-11			Increase ambulation			Increase ambulation		
PT:	Exercises per protocol / Ambulate to chair / O.T. referral, if necessary / ___ P.T. ___ O.T.			Exercises per protocol / Increase ambulation / Bathroom transfer / OT consult if necessary ___ O.T. / Start home exercise program ___ P.T.			Exercises continued / Increase ambulation / Stairs/crutches prn / ADL Instruction prm ___ O.T. ___ P.T.			Exercises continued / Increase ambulation / Stairs/crutches prn ___ P.T.		
NUTRITION	DAT: took 50% / HS Supplement ___ RN			DAT: took 75% / HS Supplement ___ RN			DAT: took 75% / HS Supplement			Advance as tol.		
SELF-CARE	1/2 bath; assist w/HS care			Advance self care as tol.			Advance self care as tol.			Advance as tol.		
ELIMINATION	*Foley; voiding qs; STOOL SOFTENER; laxative prn			*DC Foley/voiding qs; STOOL SOFT-ENER; Suppository if no BM 7-3			Voiding qs / STOOL SOFTENER			Voiding qs		
DISCHARGE PLANNING/ TEACHING	SWS evaluate discharge plan / DC date / Caregiver identified: / Reinforce hip precautions / Connections referral prn			Assess need for/order home equipment / ORIF: Discharge Instructions / ___ Mobility / ___ Meds / ___ ADL's / Discuss role of nutrition in healing			DISCHARGE ORIF patient / ENDO: Discharge Instructions / ___ Mobility / ___ Meds / ___ ADL's			Discharge endoprosthesis patient		
LAB/ DIAGNOSTICS*	PTT if on prophylaxis**			PTT if on prophylaxis**						PTT if on prophylaxis**		
	Init. Signature D E N			Init. Signature D E N			Init. Signature D E N			Init. Signature D E N		

Variance Codes
A-Not Indicated
B-Patient condition
C-Physician order override
D-Equipment/supplies
E-Pt/family decision
F-Family unavailable
G-Scheduling
H-Service not provided
I-Department closed
J-Placement availability
K-Docum. for DC
L-Physician DC plan
Z-Other

© OHMC 5/24/93   mac/xl/fhrpathway
*Physician order required
From Victor M. Goldberg, M.D., Department of Orthopedics, University Hospitals of Cleveland.

**THE BRYN MAWR HOSPITAL
NURSING DEPARTMENT**

NURSING ADMISSION ASSESSMENT

DATE __2/6/95__   TIME OF ARRIVAL __14:00__

FROM __ER__

ACCOMPANIED BY __friend__

VIA: WHEELCHAIR _____ STRETCHER __✓__ AMBULATORY _____

ID BRACELET __✓__ INFORMATION OBTAINED FROM __patient__

I. VITAL STATISTICS

TEMP __101__ PULSE __120__ RESP __30__

ORAL __✓__ RECTAL _____ AXILLARY _____

BP __140/90__ RA __143/86__ LA __138/88__ POSITION __sitting__

WEIGHT __148__ HEIGHT __5'6"__

SCALE: BED _____ CHAIR _____ STANDING __✓__

DEFERRED _____

ORIENTED TO ROOM __✓__

PROSTHESIS, APPLIANCES OR OTHER DEVICES: __0__

DENTURES __0__   *WALKER/CANE/CRUTCHES _____

FULL: UPPER __0__ LOWER __0__   *ARTIFICIAL LIMBS _____

PARTIAL: UPPER __0__ LOWER __0__   *BRACES _____

EYE GLASSES __✓__   *FALSE EYE _____

CONTACT LENSES __✓__   WIG _____

HEARING AID __0__

OTHER __0__

COMMENTS __glasses and contacts in drawer__

PATIENT HAS BROUGHT TO HOSPITAL? YES _____ NO _____

EXCEPTIONS _____

II. ALLERGIES: DRUGS __✓__ DYES _____ FOOD __✓__ OTHER _____ NONE KNOWN _____

SPECIFY AGENT	DESCRIBE REACTION (IF KNOWN)	
Keflex	Rash	
Tomatoes	Rash	

III. HEALTH PERCEPTION-HEALTH MAINTENANCE

A. PRESENT ILLNESS:

1. ADMITTING DIAGNOSIS __Diabetes R/o Kidney Infection__

2. REASON FOR ADMISSION (PATIENT'S STATEMENT) __"Fever for 4 days"__

3. DURATION OF PRESENT ILLNESS __4 days__

4. PAST AND PRESENT TREATMENT OF PRESENT ILLNESS AND RESPONSE __None__

5. PATIENT AWARE OF DIAGNOSIS: YES __✓__ NO _____ NOT ESTABLISHED _____

B. PREVIOUS ILLNESSES: (INCLUDING HOSPITALIZATION)

__Multiple admissions for diabetic control and
urinary tract infections__

8183 PG 1 (REV 9/90)

C. ARE YOU TAKING ANY MEDICATIONS (PRESCRIBED OR OVER THE COUNTER) YES ✓ NO _____

MEDICATION	DOSE	WHEN DO YOU TAKE IT	WHY DO YOU TAKE IT	LAST DOSE	BROUGHT TO HOSPITAL YES	BROUGHT TO HOSPITAL NO	DISPOSITION
Tylenol	500mg	PRN	Fever/Aches	12:00		✓	—
Regular Insulin	5u	AC	Diabetes	8:00		✓	—

D. DO YOU OR HAVE YOU EVER USED?

	YES	NO	LAST USED	FREQUENCY/AMOUNT
ALCOHOL		✓		
RECREATIONAL DRUGS		✓		

E. DO YOU SMOKE? YES _____ PKS/DAY _____ HOW LONG _____ _____

NO: DID YOU EVER SMOKE? NO ✓ YES ____ PKS/DAY _____ HOW LONG _____ WHEN DID YOU QUIT _____

IV. COGNITIVE PERCEPTUAL: HEADACHE _yes_ SEIZURES _0_ BLACKOUTS _0_ DIZZINESS _0_ NO C/O _—_

A. LEVEL OF CONSCIOUSNESS: ALERT _✓_ DROWSY _____ RESPONDS TO: PAIN _____ VERBAL STIMULI _____ UNRESPONSIVE _____

B. ORIENTED: TIME _✓_ PLACE _✓_ PERSON _✓_ COMMENTS _—_____

C. MOOD: RELAXED _____ ANXIOUS _✓_ SAD _____ ANGRY _____ WITHDRAWN _____ OTHER _____

D. RECENT MEMORY CHANGE: YES _____ NO _✓_ SPECIFY _____

E. RESPONDS TO DIRECTIONS: YES _✓_ NO _____ SPECIFY _____

F. SPEECH: CLEAR _✓_ SLURRED _____ GARBLED _____ UNABLE TO SPEAK _____ APHASIC _____

G. LANGUAGE SPOKEN: ENGLISH _✓_ OTHER _____

H. HEARING: WNL _✓_ IMPAIRED _____ CORRECTED _____ DEAF _____ SIGN LANGUAGE _____ LIP READS _____

I. VISION: WNL _✓_ IMPAIRED _____ CORRECTED _✓_ BLIND _____

J. PAIN: YES _✓_ NO _____ DESCRIBE _headache, right flank pain_____

HOW DO YOU MANAGE YOUR PAIN? _Tylenol_____

K. LEARNING READINESS: NO LIMITATIONS _____ WILLING TO LEARN _✓_ RESISTS LEARNING _____

EMOTIONALLY READY TO LEARN: YES _✓_ NO _____ REQUIRES CONCRETE LANGUAGE/REINFORCEMENT _____ FORGETFUL _____

TEACHING TO BE DIRECTED PRIMARILY TO _patient_____
FAMILY MEMBER/SIGNIFICANT OTHER

L. COMMENTS _Knowledgeable about diabetes_____

V. ROLE RELATIONSHIP (PSYCHOSOCIAL) / DISCHARGE PLANNING

A. OCCUPATION _Teacher_____

B. LIVE ALONE _✓_ WITH FAMILY _____ NURSING HOME _____ OTHER _____ COMMENT _____

C. DESCRIBE PHYSICAL ENVIRONMENT _2 story house_____

D. ANTICIPATED DISCHARGE TO: ECF _____ HOME CARE SERVICES _____

OTHER _____ HOME _✓_ IF GOING HOME, WHO COULD HELP YOU WITH

HEALTHCARE NEEDS AFTER DISCHARGE? _friends_____

E. DO YOU WISH TO SEE A MEMBER OF THE CLERGY WHILE YOU ARE HERE? YES _____ NO _✓_ AFFILIATION _____

F. COMMENTS _____

VI. HEALTH HISTORY/ASSESSMENT

A. CARDIOVASCULAR: ANGINA _0_ ARRHYTHMIA _0_ MURMUR _0_ EDEMA _0_ PALPITATIONS _0_

CHEST PAIN _0_ MI _0_ CVA _0_ ANEURYSM _0_ HYPERTENSION _✓_

PACEMAKER _0_ TYPE _0_ NO C/O _____

PULSE: STRONG _✓_ WEAK _____ REGULAR _✓_ IRREGULAR _____

RIGHT DORSALIS PEDAL PULSE: STRONG _✓_ WEAK _____ ABSENT _____

LEFT DORSALIS PEDAL PULSE: STRONG _✓_ WEAK _____ ABSENT _____

COMMENTS _____

8183 PG 2 (REV 9/90)

B. RESPIRATORY: COUGH __0__ PRODUCTIVE __0__ PAIN __0__ DESCRIBE __0_____

FREQUENT COLDS _0_ HOARSENESS _0_ ASTHMA _0_ TB _0_ SOB: ON EXERTION _0_ AT REST _0_ NO C/O __✓__

COMMENTS _____

C. RENAL: KIDNEY STONES __✓__ INFECTIONS ____ RETENTION __✓__ BURNING __✓__ POLYURIA __✓__ DYSURIA _____ NO C/O____

URINARY DEVICES? __0__ TYPE __0_____

INCONTINENCE __0__ DAYTME __0__ NOCTURNAL __0__ STRESS __0__

DO YOU GET UP DURING NIGHT TO URINATE? YES __✓__ NO _____

COMMENTS __Probable Kidney infection_____

D. GASTROINTESTINAL (NUTRITION/METABOLIC)

1. HISTORY OF DIABETES? YES __✓__ NO ____ DO YOU TEST FOR SUGAR? YES __✓__ NO ____ URINE ____ BLOOD __✓__

DIET CONTROLLED _____ INSULIN DEPENDENT __✓__ ORAL HYPOGLYCEMICS _____

NUMBER OF YEARS __10__ PREVIOUS DIABETES EDUCATION: YES __✓__ NO _____

2. NUMBER OF MEALS/DAY __3__ SNACKS __2__ SPECIAL DIET __0_____

3. PATIENT'S ABILITY TO EAT: INDEPENDENT __✓__ WITH ASSISTANCE __0__ SPECIFY __0_____

DIFFICULTY SWALLOWING __0__

4. WEIGHT CHANGE IN THE LAST SIX MONTHS: NONE __0__ LOST _____ LBS GAINED _____ LBS

5. DO YOU EXPERIENCE NAUSEA/VOMITING? YES __✓__ NO _____ RELATED TO __fever_____

6. DO YOU EXPERIENCE CRAMPING __0__ HEARTBURN __0__ RECTAL PAIN __0__ GAS __0__ LAST BM: __yesterday__

7. BOWEL: USUAL TIME: __10__ A.M. _____ P.M. FREQUENCY: DAILY _____ EVERY OTHER DAY __✓__ OTHER _____

INCONTINENCE __0__ DEVICES USED __0_____

COLOR: BROWN __✓__ CLAY-COLORED __0__ BLACK __0__ BLOOD __0__

CONSTIPATION: NONE _____ OCCASIONALLY __✓__ FREQUENTLY _____

DIARRHEA: NONE _____ OCCASIONALLY __✓__ FREQUENTLY _____ OSTOMY _____

LAXATIVES/ENEMAS USED/HOW OFTEN? (SPECIFY) ____0_____

8. ABDOMEN: SOFT __✓__ NON-TENDER __✓__ NON-DISTENDED _____ FIRM _____ TENDER _____ DISTENDED _____

BOWEL SOUNDS: PRESENT __✓__ ABSENT _____

COMMENTS: _____

E. SKIN CONDITION

COLOR: WNL __✓__ PALE _____ CYANOTIC _____ JAUNDICE _____ OTHER _____

TEMP: WARM __✓__ COOL _____ TURGOR: WNL _____ POOR _____

EDEMA: NO __✓__ YES _____ DESCRIPTION/LOCATION _____

LESIONS: NO __✓__ YES _____ DESCRIPTION/LOCATION _____

DECUBITUS: NO __✓__ YES _____ LOCATION(S) _____ (SEE TISSUE TRAUMA FORM)

BRUISES: NO __✓__ YES _____ DESCRIPTION/LOCATION _____

RASHES: NO __✓__ YES _____ DESCRIPTION/LOCATION _____

REDNESS: NO __✓__ YES _____ DESCRIPTION/LOCATION _____

COMMENTS: _____

F. MUSCULO-SKELETAL: CRAMPING _____ ARTHRITIS _____ STIFFNESS ✓ SWELLING _____ NO C/O _____

MOTOR FUNCTION: RIGHT ARM: WNL ✓ AMPUTATED ___ SPASTIC ___ FLACCID ___ WEAKNESS ___ PARALYSIS ___ OTHER ___

LEFT ARM: WNL ✓ AMPUTATED ___ SPASTIC ___ FLACCID ___ WEAKNESS ___ PARALYSIS ___ OTHER ___

RIGHT LEG: WNL ✓ AMPUTATED ___ SPASTIC ___ FLACCID ___ WEAKNESS ___ PARALYSIS ___ OTHER ___

LEFT LEG: WNL ✓ AMPUTATED ___ SPASTIC ___ FLACCID ___ WEAKNESS ___ PARALYSIS ___ OTHER ___

COMMENTS ___Has some joint stiffness_____

VII. SLEEP-REST/ACTIVITY

A. USUAL SLEEP PATTERN: BEDTIME _____ HOURS SLEPT _____ NAPS: NO ✓ YES _____

B. DIFFICULTY FALLING ASLEEP: NO ✓ YES _____ SPECIFY _____

C. SLEEP AIDS USED: NO ✓ YES _____ SPECIFY _____

D. DOES PATIENT HAVE DIFFICULTY/PROBLEMS IN:

BATHING: NO ✓ YES _____ SPECIFY _____

DRESSING: NO ✓ YES _____ SPECIFY _____

AMBULATING: NO ✓ YES _____ BALANCE/GAIT: STEADY _____ UNSTEADY _____ TIRES EASILY _____ WEAKNESS _____

COMMENTS ___independent_____

VIII. SEXUAL HEALTH (FEMALES)

A. LMP 2/1 LAST PAP SMEAR 10/94

B. DO YOU EXAMINE YOUR BREASTS? YES ✓ NO _____ HOW OFTEN? Every month

C. IF NO, DO YOU KNOW HOW? YES _____ NO _____ WOULD YOU BE INTERESTED IN LEARNING? YES _____ NO _____

PAMPHLET GIVEN? YES _____ NO _____ COMMENTS _____

IX. **ASSESSMENT SUMMARY:** ___Acutely ill female who manages home care well.___

X. **NURSING DIAGNOSES:** ___High Risk For Fluid Volume Deficit R/T fever and nausea.___

XI. **THE FOLLOWING SECTIONS WERE DEFERRED ON ADMISSION (IDENTIFY BY SECTION NUMBER):** ___None___

REASON: _____

DATE/TIME	COMPLETED BY		PRIMARY NURSE	DATE/TIME	REVIEWED BY PRIMARY NURSE	
2/6/95 13:00	R Alfaro	RN	YES ✓ NO ___	___/___		RN
___/___		RN	YES ___ NO ___	___/___		RN

8183 PG 4 (REV 9/90)

THE BRYN MAWR HOSPITAL NURSING DEPARTMENT

NEUROLOGICAL ASSESSMENT SHEET

Pupil size reference: 1MM · 2MM · 3MM · 4MM · 5MM · 6MM · 7MM · 8MM · 9MM

				2/12/95	2/12	2/12	2/12						
	DATE			2/12/95	2/12	2/12	2/12						
	TIME				1:00	9:00	17:00						
V I T A L S	BLOOD PRESSURE				120/70	110/70	112/68					RESPIRATORY TYPE	
	PULSE				74	80	72					N = NORMAL	
	TEMPERATURE				98	98	98					CS = CHEYNE STOKES	
	RESPIRATORY RATE				20	22	20					SH = SUSTAINED HYPERVENTILATION	
	RESPIRATORY TYPE				N	N	N						
C O M A S C A L E	EYES OPEN	SPONTANEOUSLY	4									E = EYES CLOSED BY SWELLING	
		TO COMMAND	3		✓	✓	✓						
		TO PAIN	2										
		NO RESPONSE	1										
	BEST MOTOR RESPONSE	OBEYS COMMANDS	6		✓	✓	✓					RECORD BEST ARM RESPONSE	
		LOCALIZES PAIN	5										
		FLEXION WITHDRAWAL	4										
		FLEXION (ABNORMAL)	3										
		EXTENSION (ABNORMAL)	2										
		NO RESPONSE	1										
	BEST VERBAL RESPONSE	ORIENTED	5			✓	✓					T = ENDOTRACHEAL TUBE OR TRACHEOSTOMY	
		CONFUSED	4		✓								
		INAPPROPRIATE WORDS	3										
		INCOMPREHENSIBLE SOUNDS	2									A = APHASIA	
		NO RESPONSE	1										
	TOTAL SCORE				13	14	14						
P U P I L S	SIZE		R		7	6	7					B = BRISK S = SLUGGISH	
	REACTION				S	B	B					N = NO REACTION C = CLOSED	
	SIZE		L		7	6	7					SC = SUSTAINED CONSTRICTION 2° CATARACT SURGERY	
	REACTION				B	B	B						
L I M B M O V E M E N T	GRADE LIMB SPONTANEOUS OR TO COMMAND. DO NOT RATE REFLEX MOVEMENT		RA		5	5	5					LIMB MOVEMENT SCALE 0 = PARALYSIS	
			RL		5	5	5					1 = VISIBLE MUSCLE CONTRACTION; NO MOVEMENT	
			LA		5	5	5					2 = WEAK CONTRACTION; NOT ENOUGH TO OVERCOME GRAVITY	
			LL		5	5	5						
L I M B S E N S A T I O N	DULL		RA		N	N	N					3 = MOVE AGAINST GRAVITY; NOT EXTERNAL RESISTANCE	
			RL		N	N	N					4 = NORMAL ROM; CAN BE OVERCOME BY INCREASED GRAVITY	
			LA		N	N	N					5 = NORMAL MUSCLE STRENGTH	
			LL		N	N	N					SENSATION CODES	
	SHARP		RA		N	N	N					N = NORMAL	
			RL		N	N	N					D = DECREASED	
			LA		N	N	N					A = ABSENT	
			LL		N	N	N						
	SEIZURE ACTIVITY				A	A	A					A = ABSENT P = PRESENT	
	GAG REFLEX				P	P	P					A = ABSENT P = PRESENT	
	INITIALS												

SIGNATURE	INITIALS	SIGNATURE	INITIALS
R. Alfaro RN	RA		
C. Sechrist RN	CS		
A. Carlson	AC		

F8084 (REV 1/91)

THE BRYN MAWR HOSPITAL
NURSING SERVICE

NEURO-VASCULAR ASSESSMENT FLOW SHEET

EXTREMITY(IES) TO BE ASSESSED: _Left lower leg_

FREQUENCY OF ASSESSMENT: _q8h_

TYPE OF EXTERNAL SUPPORT: _Cast_

Date	Time	Hospital Day	Post-Op Day	Limb	Color	Capillary Refill	Temp.	Edema	Sensation	Numbness & Tingling	Motion	Pulse	Proprioception	Comments	Signature
2/1/95	9:00	1	0	LE	Pink	R	W	P	P	N	P	P	P	Toes slightly edematous	R. Alfaro RN
2/1/95	17:00	1	0	✓	✓	✓	✓	A	P	A	✓	✓	✓	Moves toes well	C. Sechrist RN
2/2/95	1:00	2	1	✓	✓	✓	✓	✓	✓	✓	✓	✓	✓	Med for incisional pain	A. Carlson RN

KEY

Limb(s): Specify RUE, LUE, RLE, LLE
Color: Pink, Pale, Cyanotic
Capillary Refill: Rapid, Slow
Temperature: Warm, Cool, Cold
Edema: Absent (A), Present(P)
Sensation: Absent (A), Decreased (D), Present (P)

Numbness (N), Tingling (T): Present (P),
   Decreased (D), Absent (A)
Motion: Present (P), Decreased (D), Absent (A)
Pulses: Present (P), Absent (A)
Proprioception: Present (P), Absent (A)
NA: Not Applicable
*: See Nurses Notes

FORM 8066

161

American Nurses Association Standards for Practice

Standards of Care (Use of the Nursing Process)

Standard I   Assessment: The nurse collects client health data.

II   Diagnosis: The nurse analyzes assessment data in determining diagnoses.

III   Outcome Identification: The nurse identifies expected outcomes individualized to the client.

IV   Planning: The nurse develops a plan of care that prescribes interventions to attain expected outcomes.

V   Implementation: The nurse implements the interventions identified in the plan of care.

VI   Evaluation: The nurse evaluates the client's progress toward attainment of outcomes.

Standards of Professional Performance (Professional Behavior)

Standard I   Quality of Care: The nurse systematically evaluates the quality and effectiveness of nursing practice.

II   Performance Appraisal: The nurse evaluates his/her own nursing practice in relation to professional practice standards and relevant statutes and regulations.

III   Education: The nurse acquires and maintains current knowledge in nursing practice.

IV   Collegiality: The nurse contributes to the professional development of peers, colleagues, and others.

V   Ethics: The nurse's decisions and actions on behalf of clients are determined in an ethical manner.

VI   Collaboration: The nurse collaborates with the client, significant others, and healthcare providers in providing client care.

VII   Research: The nurse uses research findings in practice.

VIII   Resource Utilization: The nurse considers factors related to safety, effectiveness, and cost in planning and delivering client care.

Reprinted with permission from *Standards of Clinical Nursing Practice.* © 1991, American Nurses Association, Washington, DC.

American Nurses Association Code for Nurses

1. The nurse provides services with respect for human dignity and the uniqueness of the client unrestricted by considerations of social or economic status, personal attributes, or the nature of health problems.
2. The nurse safeguards the client's right to privacy by judiciously protecting information of a confidential nature.
3. The nurse acts to safeguard the client and the public when health care and safety are affected by the incompetent, unethical, or illegal practice of any person.
4. The nurse assumes responsibility and accountability for individual nursing judgments and actions.
5. The nurse maintains competence in nursing.
6. The nurse exercises informed judgment and uses individual competence and qualifications as criteria in seeking consultation, accepting responsibilities, and delegating nursing activities to others.
7. The nurse participates in activities that contribute to the ongoing development of the profession's body of knowledge.
8. The nurse participates in the profession's efforts to implement and improve standards of nursing.
9. The nurse participates in the profession's efforts to establish and maintain conditions of employment conducive to high quality nursing care.
10. The nurse participates in the profession's effort to protect the public from misinformation and misrepresentation and to maintain the integrity of nursing.
11. The nurse collaborates with members of the health professions and other citizens in promoting community and national efforts to meet the health needs of the public.

Reprinted with permission from *Code for Nurses with Interpretive Statements,* © 1985, American Nurses Association, Washington, DC.

A Patient's Bill of Rights

Introduction

Effective health care requires collaboration between patients and physicians and other health care professionals. Open and honest communication, respect for personal and professional values, and sensitivity to differences are integral to optimal patient care. As the setting for the provision of health services, hospitals must provide a foundation for understanding and respecting the rights and responsibilities of patients, their families, physicians, and other caregivers. Hospitals must ensure a health care ethic that respects the role of patients in decision making about treatment choices and other aspects of their care. Hospitals must be sensitive to cultural, racial, linguistic, religious, age, gender, and other differences as well as the needs of persons with disabilities.

The American Hospital Association presents *A Patient's Bill of Rights* with the expectation that it will contribute to more effective patient care and be supported by the hospital on behalf of the institution, its medical staff, employees, and patients. The American Hospital Association encourages health care institutions to tailor this bill of rights to their patient community by translating and/or simplifying the language of this bill of rights as may be necessary to ensure that patients and their families understand their rights and responsibilities.

A Patient's Bill of Rights was first adopted by the American Hospital Association in 1973. This revision was approved by the AHA Board of Trustees on October 21, 1992.

Reprinted with permission of the American Hospital Association, copyright 1992.

Bill of Rights*

1. The patient has the right to considerate and respectful care.
2. The patient has the right to and is encouraged to obtain from physicians and other direct care-givers relevant, current, and understandable information concerning diagnosis, treatment, and prognosis.

    Except in emergencies when the patient lacks decision-making capacity and the need for treatment is urgent, the patient is entitled to the opportunity to discuss and request information related to the specific procedures and/or treatments, the risks involved, the possible length of recuperation, and the medically reasonable alternatives and their accompanying risks and benefits.

    Patients have the right to know the identity of physicians, nurses, and others involved in their care, as well as when those involved are students, residents, or other trainees. The patient also has the right to know the immediate and long-term financial implications of treatment choices, insofar as they are known.
3. The patient has the right to make decisions about the plan of care prior to and during the course of treatment and to refuse a recommended treatment or plan

---

* These rights can be exercised on the patient's behalf by a designated surrogate or proxy decision maker if the patient lacks decision-making capacity, is legally incompetent, or is a minor.

of care to the extent permitted by law and hospital policy and to be informed of the medical consequences of this action. In case of such refusal, the patient is entitled to other appropriate care and services that the hospital provides or transfer to another hospital. The hospital should notify patients of any policy that might affect patient choice within the institution.

4. The patient has the right to have an advance directive (such as a living will, health care proxy, or durable power of attorney for health care) concerning treatment or designating a surrogate decision maker with the expectation that the hospital will honor the intent of that directive to the extent permitted by law and hospital policy.

   Health care institutions must advise patients of their rights under state law and hospital policy to make informed medical choices, ask if the patient has an advance directive, and include that information in patient records. The patient has the right to timely information about hospital policy that may limit its ability to implement fully a legally valid advance directive.

5. The patient has the right to every consideration of privacy. Case discussion, consultation, examination, and treatment should be conducted so as to protect each patient's privacy.

6. The patient has the right to expect that all communications and records pertaining to his/her care will be treated as confidential by the hospital, except in cases such as suspected abuse and public health hazards when reporting is permitted or required by law. The patient has the right to expect that the hospital will emphasize the confidentiality of this information when it releases it to any other parties entitled to review information in these records.

7. The patient has the right to review the records pertaining to his/her medical care and to have the information explained or interpreted as necessary, except when restricted by law.

8. The patient has the right to expect that, within its capacity and policies, a hospital will make reasonable response to the request of a patient for appropriate and medically indicated care and services. The hospital must provide evaluation, service, and/or referral as indicated by the urgency of the case. When medically appropriate and legally permissible, or when a patient has so requested, a patient may be transferred to another facility. The institution to which the patient is to be transferred must first have accepted the patient for transfer. The patient must also have the benefit of complete information and explanation concerning the need for, risks, benefits, and alternatives to such a transfer.

9. The patient has the right to ask and be informed of the existence of business relationships among the hospital, educational institutions, other health care providers, or payers that may influence the patient's treatment and care.

10. The patient has the right to consent to or decline to participate in proposed research studies or human experimentation affecting care and treatment or requiring direct patient involvement, and to have those studies fully explained prior to consent. A patient who declines to participate in research or experimentation is entitled to the most effective care that the hospital can otherwise provide.

11. The patient has the right to expect reasonable continuity of care when appropriate and to be informed by physicians and other caregivers of available and realistic patient care options when hospital care is no longer appropriate.

12. The patient has the right to be informed of hospital policies and practices that relate to patient care, treatment, and responsibilities. The patient has the right to be informed of available resources for resolving disputes, grievances, and conflicts, such as ethics committees, patient representatives, or other mechanisms available in the institution. The patient has the right to be informed of the hospital's charges for services and available payment methods.

The collaborative nature of health care requires that patients, or their families/surrogates, participate in their care. The effectiveness of care and patient satisfaction with the course of treatment depend, in part, on the patient's fulfilling certain responsibilities. Patients are responsible for providing information about past illnesses, hospitalizations, medications, and other matters related to health status. To participate effectively in decision making, patients must be encouraged to take responsibility for requesting additional information or clarification about their health status or treatment when they do not fully understand information and instructions. Patients are also responsible for ensuring that the health care institution has a copy of their written advance directive if they have one. Patients are responsible for informing their physicians and other caregivers if they anticipate problems in following prescribed treatment.

Patients should also be aware of the hospital's obligation to be reasonably efficient and equitable in providing care to other patients and the community. The hospital's rules and regulations are designed to help the hospital meet this obligation. Patients and their families are responsible for making reasonable accommodations to the needs of the hospital, other patients, medical staff, and hospital employees. Patients are responsible for providing necessary information for insurance claims and for working with the hospital to make payment arrangements, when necessary.

A person's health depends on much more than health care services. Patients are responsible for recognizing the impact of their life-style on their personal health.

Conclusion

Hospitals have many functions to perform, including the enhancement of health status, health promotion, and the prevention and treatment of injury and disease; the immediate and ongoing care and rehabilitation of patients; the education of health professionals, patients, and the community; and research. All these activities must be conducted with an overriding concern for the values and dignity of patients.

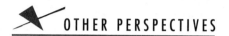

OTHER PERSPECTIVES

A Critical Thinking Model for Nursing Judgment

Merle Kataoka-Yahiro, DrPH, RN, and Coleen Saylor, PhD, RN

ABSTRACT

Increasingly, the characteristic that distinguishes a professional nurse is cognitive rather than psychomotor ability. Critical thinking is an essential component of nursing. Yet, no clear definition or conceptualization of critical thinking for nursing judgment has existed. Lack of consensus and overlapping definitions may well diminish the profession's ability to articulate this concept and facilitate its development. This article proposes the Critical Thinking Model for Nursing Judgment, which specifies five components: specific knowledge base, experience, competencies, attitudes, and standards. The model has three levels of critical thinking: basic, complex, and commitment. It provides a definition and conceptualization of critical thinking based on a review of the literature and input from nurses and nurse educators. The model provides a first step for development of further research and educational strategies to promote critical thinking as an essential part of autonomous, excellent nursing practice.

Introduction

Nurses need critical thinking in order to be safe, competent, skillful practitioners in their

Reprinted with permission from *Journal of Nursing Education*, 33(8), 351–356.

profession. The pace of knowledge development demands that nurses be critical thinkers. This article proposes the Critical Thinking Model for Nursing Judgment, which defines the concept of critical thinking as the first step toward analysis and utilization within nursing and nursing education.

Despite the interest in developing critical thinking among nurses and nursing students, few nursing studies have attempted to use a nursing critical thinking theoretical/conceptual framework. Frameworks were applied from other disciplines to nursing education (Berger, 1984; Bowers & McCarthy, 1993; Gross, Takazawa, & Rose, 1987; Jones & Brown, 1991). Miller and Malcolm (1990) alone have adapted and developed a critical thinking framework in nursing curricula evaluation. Nursing lacks a critical thinking framework that is domain-specific and encompasses all areas of nursing. The Miller and Malcolm framework contains the general components of attitude, knowledge, skill, and levels of critical thinking. The Critical Thinking Model for Nursing Judgment builds upon the concepts of Miller and Malcolm, but expands to include components of nursing experience, competencies, and standards.

The National League for Nursing (NLN) recognizes the inclusion of critical thinking as a specific criterion for the accreditation of baccalaureate programs. The criterion states: "The curriculum emphasizes the development of critical thinking and of progressively independent decision-making" (NLN, 1989). Therefore, faculty need an understandable, workable, yet comprehensive definition of critical thinking. In addition, staff developers must meet hospital accreditation standards requiring critical thinking as part of clinical competencies and, therefore, are faced with similar concerns.

Since nursing is faced with facilitating and measuring the critical thinking process in direct relationship to nursing, a domain-specific critical thinking definition is necessary. Many definitions of critical thinking exist (Ennis, 1962, 1985; Facione, 1984; Glaser, 1941; Kurfiss, 1988; McPeck, 1981; Paul, 1993; Siegel, 1980). However, there is a lack of agreement on the meaning of the concept; it is neither clearly understood nor systematically applied. The current definitions originate principally from philosophy and education and may not always be relevant to a practice discipline such as nursing. The lack of consensus and its relevancy to nursing impedes nurse educators who struggle with professional curricula and accreditation expectations to define and measure critical thinking in their curricula.

In nursing education, critical thinking has been narrowly defined as a rational-linear problem-solving activity that reflects the nursing process (Jones & Brown, 1991). Critical thinking has also been described simply as the scientific process (Kemp, 1985; Malek, 1986). Yet, it is a mistake to define critical thinking in nursing only as problem solving, scientific methodology, or nursing process because it may encompass the interaction of all of these and more.

Based on a broader, multidimensional focus within *nursing* and adapted from Ennis (1985) and Kurfiss (1988), our proposed model defines critical thinking as follows: "The critical thinking process is reflective and reasonable thinking about nursing problems without a single solution and is focused on deciding what to believe and do." The definition provides the foundation for the model (see Figure).

The impetus to create the Critical Thinking Model for Nursing Judgment stemmed from an interest in incorporating critical thinking into a new undergraduate curriculum. The model was initially influenced by Miller and Malcolm's (1990) adaptation of Glaser's (1941) definition and research on critical thinking. Glaser suggested that attitudes, knowledge, and skills influence critical thinking. Miller and Malcolm illustrated the interaction of attitudes, knowledge, and skills in the resulting levels of critical thinking attained in nursing curricula. Primary goals in the construction of the model were (a) to build upon the works

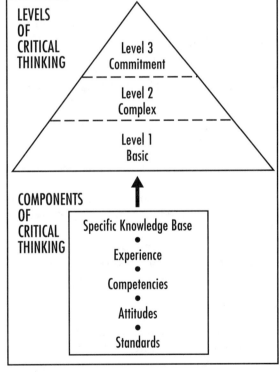

Figure
Critical Thinking Model for Nursing Judgment. Copyright 1993. Adapted from Glaser (1941), Miller and Malcolm (1990), Paul (1993), and Perry (1970).

of Glaser and Miller and Malcolm, (b) to expand the model to include other components of critical thinking believed to be domain-specific or related to nursing, and (c) to broaden the audience beyond nurse educators and nursing students to include the entire discipline of nursing.

Development of the Model

Early versions of the Critical Thinking Model for Nursing Judgment were presented to focus groups for critique of face validity. In order to be meaningful, the model must be relevant to nursing education and to practicing nurses in a variety of clinical settings; therefore, the focus groups provided feedback on clarity and relevance.

The first focus group of three nursing educators interested in critical thinking met with the authors. This group worked principally on components of the model, creating a taxonomy of the multiple terms and phrases in the current literature relative to critical thinking in nursing and in other disciplines. Specifically, this group attempted to clarify what specific competencies were unique to nursing and to clarify the relationships among terms such as the scientific process, hypothesis generation, problem solving, decision making, diagnostic reasoning, clinical inferences, clinical decision making, and nursing process. The authors synthesized their comments for a new draft of the model.

The new draft was presented to 30 practicing registered nurses enrolled in a graduate-level nursing education program. These nurses focused principally on the levels of critical thinking and validated the levels with examples from their clinical specialties. They made design suggestions, reaffirmed the existing component section of the model, and added experience as a new component. Following another series of refinements integrating these changes, a graphic design consultant made suggestions regarding the visual repre-

sentation. Finally, the initial group of nursing educators gave input for minor changes and validated this final version of the model.

Critical Thinking and Nursing Judgment

The model defines the outcome of critical thinking as nursing judgment (discipline-specific clinical judgment). That is, the outcome is the clinical judgment of nurses relevant to nursing problems in a variety of settings.

Nursing judgment entails decisions formed in direct, semi-direct, and indirect nursing care roles. As examples of these roles, staff nurses make decisions about patient care (direct), directors of nursing in agencies make decisions about distribution of nursing resources (semi-direct), and nurse educators make curricular decisions (indirect).

In contrast, clinical judgment has been defined exclusively in direct care situations. In the literature, clinical judgment is discussed more than nursing judgment (Kintgen-Andrews, 1991; Westfall, Tanner, Putzier, & Padrick, 1986). Tanner (1983) defines clinical judgment as including (a) decisions regarding what to observe in the patient situation, (b) inferential decisions, deriving meaning from data observed, and (c) decisions regarding actions that should be taken that will be of optimal benefit to the patient. Research studies have been unable to show consistently a significant relationship between clinical judgment and critical thinking. Many research studies have reported that no identifiable relationship exists between clinical judgment and critical thinking (Brooks & Shepherd, 1990; Frederickson & Mayer, 1977; Pardue, 1987). However, this may be due to the lack of refinement in design and instrumentation rather than a lack of relationship between critical thinking and clinical judgment.

The authors believe that this model provides a foundation from which relationships between variables such as critical thinking and clinical judgment can be tested and validated. The five components of critical thinking for nursing judgment are specific knowledge, experience, competencies, attitudes, and standards in nursing (see Table).

Specific Knowledge

The first component is specific *knowledge* and was based on one of Glaser's (1941) three composites of knowledge, attitudes, and skills. Glaser stated that knowledge is required in critical thinking. Others have documented the importance of domain-specific knowledge to successful clinical reasoning (Elstein, Shulman, & Sprafka, 1990). A specific knowledge base in nursing provides the data for the various critical thinking processes.

One cannot identify appropriate actions for unexpected clinical symptoms, for example,

---

TABLE
Components of
Critical Thinking in Nursing

I. Specific Knowledge Base in Nursing
II. Experience in Nursing
III. Critical Thinking Competencies
    A. General Critical Thinking Competencies
    B. Specific Critical Thinking Competencies
       in Clinical Situations
    C. Specific Critical Thinking Competency
       in Nursing
IV. Attitudes for Critical Thinking

A. Confidence	G. Perseverance
B. Independence	H. Creativity
C. Fairness	I. Curiosity
D. Responsibility	J. Integrity
E. Risk taking	K. Humility
F. Discipline	

V. Standards for Critical Thinking
    1. Intellectual Standards

A. Clear	H. Logical
B. Precise	I. Deep
C. Specific	J. Broad
D. Accurate	K. Complete
E. Relevant	L. Significant
F. Plausible	M. Adequate (for purpose)
G. Consistent	N. Fair

    2. Professional Standards
       A. Ethical criteria for nursing judgment
       B. Criteria for evaluation
       C. Professional responsibility

---

without understanding the physiology involved. Knowledge based on courses in the sciences, humanities, and nursing is necessary to think about nursing problems. The urgent need for critical thinking processes within schools and clinical settings must not obscure the basic requirement that nurses be able to access the necessary knowledge base on which to build critical thinking.

Experience

The second component is *experience*. Development of critical thinking can be limited by the lack of practical experience and opportunity to actually make decisions. Benner (1984) states that practical knowledge in an applied discipline is only developed through clinical experience. Tanner, Benner, Chesla, and Gordon (1993) describe the importance of experiential knowledge, as separate from formalized knowledge, as the "know-how that allows for the instantaneous recognition of patterns and intuitive responses" in expert judgment (p. 274). Studies of other practice disciplines also demonstrate the importance of experience (Dreyfus & Dreyfus, 1986; Schon, 1983).

The expert nurse understands the context of the situation, recognizes cues, and interprets them as relevant or irrelevant (Benner, 1984). Understanding of a complex situation only comes through experience with analysis of similar and contrasting situations. Furthermore, real world experiences provide a potent strategy to decrease simplistic thinking (Kurfiss, 1988).

Competencies

The third component is *competencies* and originates from Glaser's (1941) composite ability, *skill*. However, this model uses the word competencies to emphasize that these are cognitive rather than psychomotor processes. The competencies are of three types, based on feedback from the focus group and the review of literature. The three types of competencies are:

(1) general critical thinking competencies, (2) specific critical thinking competencies in clinical situations, and (3) specific critical thinking competency in nursing. The examples within the areas of general critical thinking competencies, specific critical thinking competencies in clinical situations, and specific critical thinking competency in nursing involve elements common to each other.

General critical thinking competencies are not unique to nursing per se, but are used in other disciplines and nonclinical situations. Examples of general critical thinking competencies are scientific process, hypothesis generation, problem solving, and decision making. The literature is replete with multiple definitions of these sometimes overlapping competencies (Brooks & Shepherd, 1990; del Bueno, 1983; Fredrickson & Mayer, 1977; Hughes & Young, 1992; Jenkins, 1985; Kurfiss, 1988; Nehring, Durham, & Macek, 1986; Pardue, 1987; Schaefer, 1974; Tanner, 1983; Wilkinson, 1992).

The next category of critical thinking competencies is found in clinical situations, both in nursing and other clinical disciplines. These processes are used by physicians and allied health professions as well as nurses. This category of clinical critical thinking competencies includes examples such as diagnostic reasoning, clinical inferences, and clinical decision making (Elstein, Shulman, & Sprafka, 1978; Tanner, Padrick, Westfall, & Putzier, 1987; Thiele, Baldwin, Hyde, Sloan, & Strandquist, 1986; Westfall et al., 1986).

The final category is the critical thinking competency specific to nursing-the nursing process. The model suggests that the nursing process is not an all-encompassing competency, but only one of the competencies of critical thinking. The format for the nursing process is unique to the discipline of nursing, just as other subject areas have disciplined ways of thinking. The nursing process provides a systematic, rational method of planning, providing, and evaluating nursing care using higher order thinking processes (Kozier, Erb, & Blais, 1992). This particular format provides a common language and process by which nurses "think through" clients' clinical problems. It provides a systematic and structural framework for nursing care (Miller & Malcolm, 1990).

In the nursing literature, some authors say that the nursing process constrains the process of critical thinking. Jones and Brown (1991) suggest that the nursing process may impede the profession's development as a legitimate science since it may not include the complex thinking processes involved in nursing practice. Miller and Malcolm (1990) criticize the nursing process for deemphasizing the contextual basis for nursing practice. Similarly, Allen, Bowers, and Diekelmann (1989) suggest that the nursing process represents an outline to organize information gathered elsewhere, "rather than a process by which to make discoveries and learn to manage that previously obtained information" (p. 9).

These three areas of competencies are not mutually exclusive, but interact to support and reinforce one another. For example, using the nursing process involves problem solving and decision making (Malek, 1986; Nehring et al., 1986; Pardue, 1987; Schaefer, 1974). Diagnostic reasoning and clinical inference are influenced by data acquisition, diagnostic accuracy, decision making, and hypothesis generation (Elstein et al., 1978; Tanner et al., 1987; Thiele et al., 1986; Westfall et al., 1986).

Attitudes for Critical Thinking

The fourth component of critical thinking is *attitudes*. This component was adapted from Glaser (1941) and the attitudinal traits were adapted from the work done by Paul (1993). Paul calls these "traits of the mind" and reminds us that they are central rather than peripheral aspects of a critical thinker. He says that if one does not persevere at reasoning, or is not fair in weighing evidence for an opposing viewpoint, or does not value curiosity or discipline, critical thinking is not possible. Similarly, independence, confidence, and responsibility are essential to arrive at one's own judgment (Paul, 1993). He mentions that integrity and humility help to acknowledge the limitations of personal knowledge or viewpoint. Creativity and risk taking may well be necessary to generate alternative and innovative viewpoints. Therefore, the ability to think critically in this model includes confidence, independence, fairness, responsibility, risk taking, discipline, perseverance, creativity, curiosity, integrity, and humility.

Standards

The fifth component, *standards*, includes two parts: intellectual standards and professional standards. The model adopts Paul's (1993) intellectual standards and expands this section to include professional standards specific to nursing. Paul states that critical thinking must meet universal intellectual standards. Paul says that in comparing and evaluating the critical thinking ability of individuals, one should apply the following intellectual standards: clarity, precision, specificity, accuracy, relevancy, plausibility, consistency, logicality, depth, broadness, completeness, significance, adequacy, and fairness.

The professional standards section is necessary for critical thinking in nursing. It sets precedence in requiring nurses to use critical thinking for the good of individuals or groups rather than to cause harm or undermine the situation. The professional standards section includes ethical criteria for nursing judgment (i.e., ANA's Code for Nurses with Interpretive Statements), criteria for evaluation (i.e., NLN accreditation or JCAHO accreditation), and criteria for professional responsibility (i.e., Nurse Practice Act or ANA Standards of Practice).

Levels of Critical Thinking in Nursing

The model identifies three levels of critical thinking in nursing: basic, complex, and commitment. These are adapted from Perry's (1970) "positions" of the ability to think critically, which describe a scheme for intellectual and ethical development. Perry's scheme may be seen in three parts, each consisting of three "positions."

In the first part, the self sees answers as dichotomous (dualism) and assumes that the authorities have the right answers for every problem. Also included in the first part are the multiplicity positions in which diversity of opinions and values among the authorities is acceptable.

In the second part, relativism, the self continues to recognize the diversity of individual outlook and perception, but the self rather than the authority is the prime mover of this process. The self has the ability to detach, analyze, and examine alternatives systematically.

In the third part, commitment, the self anticipates the necessity of personal choices in a relativistic world after the relative merits of the alternatives have been examined. In our model, the basic level is adapted from Perry's (1970) dualism position, the complex level from Perry's multiplicity and relativism positions, and the commitment level from Perry's commitment positions.

Basic

At this level, answers to complex problems are right or wrong, and one right answer usually exists for each complex problem. This level is an early step in the development of reasoning ability in each particular area of nursing. Unfamiliar content, inexperience, inadequate competencies, inappropriate attitudes, and nonutilization of standards can restrict personal ability to move to higher levels, although the goal is to think on a higher level than basic.

Complex

At this level, the nurse's best answer to a problem may be, "It depends." Nurses at this level realize that alternative, perhaps conflicting, solutions exist, each with benefits and costs. Unique aspects of the client and the context matter in weighing alternative answers. A common example of the need for complex thinking is the consideration of deviation from standard protocols or rules when complex client situations have to be taken into account. Nurses at this level may find that there is not one normal pattern; rather, accurate assessment may depend on salient situational features. At this level there may be more than one solution, but the nurse has not made a commitment to any one solution.

Commitment

At the complex level, one may be aware of the complexities of alternative solutions, yet defer from commitment to any one of the solutions. At the commitment level, however, the nurse chooses an action or belief based on the alternatives identified at the complex level.

However, an action may be delayed until a later time. For example, initially, a staff nurse may override a learned racial bias to accept a belief from a more egalitarian position. This belief will eventually result in the nurses's advocacy for improved access to health care for people of all races. If that chosen action is unsuccessful, alternative solutions are considered and utilized.

Although there are times when a nurse functions at the basic level, the goal is to reach the commitment level. Like Perry's (1970) positions of critical thinking, the levels of critical thinking in this model reflect a developmental approach. The model suggests that critical thinking ability moves up and down the hierarchy of levels, depending on the nurse, but commitment is the ultimate goal.

Assumptions

The nursing environment provides the context that constrains or facilitates critical thinking. Nurses are faced with increased workloads, and nursing students are often reinforced for memorizing and retaining factual information. In such environments, nurses and nursing students are impeded in developing their critical thinking abilities. Characteristics of a work or learning environment conducive to critical thinking are flexibility, creativity, support for change, and risk taking. If a climate of intellectual openness and integrity in the classroom or agency is lacking, critical thinking can be stifled at the outset (Paul, 1984). Similarly, environments that demand perfection or reinforce the status quo constrain the critical thinking climate necessary among colleagues for excellent nursing judgment. If new ideas are not exchanged and sometimes accepted, then why think through a troublesome nursing situation or an outdated protocol?

In addition to environment, individual characteristics influence one's critical thinking ability. Age, culture, gender, ethnicity, socioeconomic status, intelligence, and level of development may affect the components of critical thinking, which in turn influence one's level of critical thinking.

Summary

Today's increasingly complex health care environment creates an urgency for professionals to be able to solve complex problems. The Model of Critical Thinking for Nursing Judgment provides a definition and conceptualization of this process based on the literature and critique from nurses and nurse educators. The model includes five components of critical thinking: specific knowledge base, experience, competencies, attitudes, and standards. These components influence the three levels of critical thinking: basic, complex, and commitment.

The model underscores the view that the nursing process alone is not an adequate conceptualization of critical thinking. Other processes are needed for nursing judgment. Nursing educators and staff developers must ask themselves whether nursing programs are socializing nurses to think at a basic level. The hierarchy of levels reminds us that the objective in complex nursing situations is the commitment level, rather than being satisfied with simple answers to complicated situations.

The model may provide a basis for future research and educational strategies. The components and levels can be used by researchers to develop reliable and valid instruments, operationalize definitions, and examine relationships within the model. In addition, the model will provide nurse educators with a framework for developing teaching strategies and assessing students' potential for critical thinking. Finally, this conceptualization lays a foundation for nurses and nurse educators to promote critical thinking abilities within nursing. Further discussion of the model is essential to facilitate the understanding of the critical thinking process.

References

Allen, D., Bowers, B., & Diekelmann, N. (1989). Writing to learn: A reconceptualization of thinking and writing in the nursing curriculum. Journal of Nursing Education, 28, 6-11.

Benner, P. (1984). From novice to expert: Excellence and power in clinical practice. Menlo Park, CA: Addison-Wesley.

Berger, M. (1984). Clinical thinking ability and nursing students. Journal of Nursing Education, 23, 306-308.

Bowers, B., & McCarthy, D. (1993). Developing analytic thinking skills in early undergraduate education. Journal of Nursing Education, 32, 107-114.

Brooks, K., & Shepherd, J. (1990). The relationship between clinical decision-making skills in nursing and general critical thinking abilities of senior nursing students in four types of nursing programs. Journal of Nursing Education, 29, 391-399.

del Bueno, D. (1983). Doing the right thing: Nurses' ability to make clinical decisions. Nurse Educator, 8, 7-11.

Dreyfus, H., & Dreyfus, S. (1986). Mind over machine. New York: Free Press

Elstein, A., Shulman, L., & Sprafka, S. (1978). Medical problem-solving: An analysis of clinical reasoning. Cambridge, MA: Harvard University Press.

Elstein, A., Shulman, L., & Sprafka, S. (1990). Medical problem-solving: A ten-year retrospective. Evaluation and the Health Professions, 13, 5-86.

Ennis, R. (1962). A concept of critical thinking: A proposed basis for research in the teaching and evaluation of critical thinking ability. Harvard Educational Review, 32, 81-111.

Ennis, R. (1985). A logical basis for measuring critical thinking skills. Educational Leadership, 43, 45-48.

Facione, P. (1984). Toward a theory of critical thinking. Liberal Education, 70, 253-261.

Frederickson, K, & Mayer, G. (1977). Problem-solving skills: What effect does education have? American Journal of Nursing, 77, 1167-1169.

Glaser, E. (1941). An experiment in the development of critical thinking. New York: Bureau of Publications, Teachers College, Columbia University.

Gross, Y., Takazawa, E., & Rose, C. (1987). Critical thinking and nursing education. Journal of Nursing Education, 26, 317-323.

Hughes, K., & Young, W. (1992). Decision making: Stability of clinical decisions. Nurse Educator, 17(3), 12-16.

Jenkins, H. (1985). Improving clinical decision making in nursing. Journal of Nursing Education, 24, 242-243.

Jones, S., & Brown, L. (1991). Critical thinking: Impact on nursing education. Journal of Advanced Nursing, 16, 529-533.

Kemp, V. (1985). Concept analysis as a strategy for promoting critical thinking. Journal of Nursing Education, 24, 382-384.

Kintgen-Andrews, J. (1991). Critical thinking and nursing education: Perplexities and insights. Journal of Nursing Education, 30, 152-157.

Kozier, B., Erb, G., & Blais, K. (1992). Concepts and issues in nursing practice. (2nd ed.). Redwood City, CA: Addison-Wesley.

Kurfiss, J. (1988). Critical thinking: Theory, research, practice and possibilities. ASHE-ERIC Higher Education Report No. 2. Washington, DC: Association for the Study of Higher Education.

Malek, C. (1986). A model for teaching critical thinking. Nurse Educator, 11(6), 20-23.

McPeck, J. (1981). Critical thinking and education. New York: St. Martin's Press.

Miller, M., & Malcolm, N. (1990). Critical thinking in the nursing curriculum. Nursing and Health Care, 11, 67-73.

National League for Nursing. (1989). Criterion for the evaluation of baccalaureate and higher degree programs in nursing (6th ed.). New York: Author.

Nehring, W., Durham, J., & Macek, M. (1986). Effective teaching: A problem-solving paradigm. Nurse Educator, 11(3), 23-26.

Pardue, S. (1987). Decision-making skills and critical thinking ability among associate degree, diploma, baccalaureate, and master's prepared nurses. Journal of Nursing Education, 26, 354-361.

Paul, R. (1984). Critical thinking: Fundamental to education for a free society. Educational Leadership, 42, 4-14.

Paul, R. (1993). The art of redesigning instruction. In J. Willsen & A.J.A. Binker (Eds.), Critical thinking: How to prepare students for a rapidly changing world (p. 319). Santa Rosa, CA: Foundation for Critical Thinking.

Perry, W. (1970). Forms of intellectual and ethical development in the college years: A scheme. New York: Holt, Rinehart & Winston.

Schaefer, J. (1974). The interrelatedness of decision. American Journal of Nursing, 74, 1852-1856.

Schon, D. (1983). The reflective practitioner. New York: Basic Books.

Siegel, H. (1980). Critical thinking as an educational ideal. The Educational Reform, XLV, 7-23.

Tanner, C. (1983). Research on clinical judgment. In W. Holzemer (Ed.), Review of research in nursing education (pp. 1-32), Thorofare, NJ: Charles B. Slack.

Tanner, C., Benner, P., Chesla, C., & Gordon, D. (1993). The phenomenology of knowing the patient. Image: Journal of Nursing Scholarship, 25, 273-280.

Tanner, C., Padrick, K., Westfall, U., & Putzier, D. (1987). Diagnostic reasoning strategies of nurses and nursing students. Nursing Research, 36, 358-363.

Thiele, J., Baldwin, J., Hyde, R., Sloan, B., & Strandquist, G. (1986). An investigation of decision theory: What are the effects of teaching cue recognition? Journal of Nursing Education, 25, 319-324.

Westfall, U., Tanner, C., Putzier, D., & Padrick K. (1986). Activating clinical inferences: A component of diagnostic reasoning in nursing. Research in Nursing and Health, 9, 269-277.

Wilkinson, J. (1992). Nursing process in action: A critical thinking approach. Redwood City, CA: Addison-Wesley.

ADVANCED PRACTICE NURSE A nurse who, by virtue of credentials (usually completion of a masters program and certification), has a wide scope of authority to act (may include treating medical problems and prescribing medications).

AIR EMBOLISM An air bubble that gets into the blood stream. Can be fatal.

ANALYSIS A mental process in which one seeks to get a better understanding of the nature of something by carefully separating the whole into smaller parts. For example, if you want to know more about someone's physical health, you examine each organ and system separately.

ANAPHYLACTIC SHOCK Extreme hypotension caused by an allergic reaction; requires immediate treatment, or can be fatal.

ASSESSMENT TOOL A printed form used to ensure that key information is gathered and recorded during assessment.

ASSUMPTION Something that's taken for granted without proof. (Compare with *Hypothesis* and *Inference*.)

ATTITUDE A way of acting, feeling, or thinking that shows one's disposition, opinion, etc. (e.g., "a threatening attitude").

BASELINE DATA Information that describes the status of a problem before treatment begins.

BEHAVIOR The way in which someone acts, reacts, or functions.

CARING BEHAVIOR Behavior that shows understanding and respect for another's perceptions, feelings, needs, and desires.

CIRCUMSTANCES The conditions or facts attending an event or having some bearing on it.

CLASSIFY To arrange or group together data according to categories, thereby increasing understanding because relationships become more obvious.

CLIENT-CENTERED GOAL A statement or phrase that details what the client or patient is expected to be able to do when the plan of care is terminated. For example, "Will be discharged home able to walk independently using a walker by 8/24."

CLIENT-CENTERED OUTCOME See *Client-centered goal.*

CLINICAL JUDGMENT A term used for critical thinking in the clinical area (as compared with critical thinking in the classroom). Usually involves a series of clinical decisions that include: (1) deciding what to observe, (2) deciding what data suggest (drawing conclusions about the diagnosis), and (3) deciding what actions to take (Tanner, 1983).

CLINICAL REASONING See *Clinical judgment.*

COLLABORATIVE ACTIONS Nursing actions prescribed by a physician or facility protocol. For example, administering IV's. (Compare with *Independent actions*.)

COLLABORATIVE PROBLEM An actual or potential problem with structure or function of an organ or system requiring nurse-prescribed and physician-prescribed interventions.

COMPETENCE The quality of having the necessary knowledge, skill, and attitude to perform an action.

CONTEXT The circumstances in which a particular event occurs.

CRITICAL Characterized by careful and exact evaluation; crucial.

CRITICAL PATH A standard plan of care for a particular medical problem that has been developed through professional consensus (nursing, medicine, other key health care professionals). The purpose of the critical path is to provide a guide to set daily priorities, in order to expedite care delivery. See page 155 for an example of critical path.

CUES See *Data*.

DATA Pieces of information about health status (e.g., vital signs).

DATA BASE ASSESSMENT Comprehensive data collected when the client first enters the health care facility to gain information about all aspects of the health status.

DATA BASE FORM See *Assessment tool*.

DEFINING CHARACTERISTICS The signs and symptoms usually associated with a specific nursing diagnosis.

DEFINITIVE DIAGNOSIS The most specific, most correct diagnosis.

DEFINITIVE INTERVENTIONS The most specific actions required to prevent, resolve, or control a health problem.

DIAGNOSE To make a judgment and identify and name a problem or strength after careful analysis of evidence from an assessment.

DIAGNOSTIC ERROR When a health problem has been overlooked or incorrectly identified.

DIAGNOSTIC REASONING A method of thinking that involves specific, deliberate use of critical thinking to reach conclusions about health status.

DIAGNOSTIC STATEMENT A phrase that clearly describes a diagnosis; includes the problem name, related (risk) factors, and any evidence confirming the diagnosis.

DIAPHORETIC The condition of being sweaty, usually suspected to be a sign of a health problem (e.g., shock, disease).

DEDUCTIVE REASONING Drawing *specific* conclusions from *general* principles and rules. For example: "Since it's true that bacteria are killed by antibiotics, Jane's bacterial infection requires treatment with antibiotics." (Compare with *Inductive* reasoning.)

DISPOSITION One's customary frame of mind or manner of response.

DIURETIC A drug given to enhance kidney function, thereby increasing fluid elimination from the body.

EFFICIENCY The quality of being able to produce a desired effect safely, with minimal risks, expense, and unnecessary effort.

EMBOLI More than one embolus. (See *Embolus*.)

EMBOLUS A clot that has moved through one vessel and lodged in another, reducing or totally blocking blood supply to tissues usually nourished by the vessels involved. (Compare with *Thrombus*.)

EMPATHY Understanding another's feelings or perceptions, but not sharing the same feelings or point of view. (Compare with *Sympathy*.)

EMPIRIC Relying solely on practical experience, ignoring science.

EPIDEMIOLOGY The body of knowledge reflecting what is known about a specific health state.

ESTHETICS A sense of what is pleasing to the eye.

ETHICS The study of the general nature of morals and of the specific moral choices to be made by individuals in relationships with others.

ETIOLOGY The cause or contributing factors of a health problem.

EVALUATION The fifth step of the nursing process, during which the extent of goal achievement is determined; each of the previous four steps is analyzed to identify factors that enhanced or hindered progress, and the plan of care is modified or terminated as indicated.

EXPECTED OUTCOME See *C*lient-centered outcome.

FOCUS ASSESSMENT Data collection that aims to gain specific information about only one aspect of health status.

GUIDELINES Documents that delineate how care is to be provided in specific situations.

HABIT A pattern of behavior that is set by continual repetition, and therefore usually done easily even without thought.

HABITS OF INQUIRY Habits that enhance the ability to search for the truth (e.g., following rules of logic).

HIGH-RISK DIAGNOSIS A diagnosis for which someone is more at risk than others in the same situation. For example, anyone on prolonged bed rest has a potential (risk) for skin breakdown. However, an elderly diabetic is more at risk for skin breakdown than others on prolonged bed rest.

HIGH-RISK PROBLEM See *H*igh-risk diagnosis.

HUMAN RESPONSES Reactions of individuals or groups to health care concerns. For example, someone may react to being told they are diabetic by feeling overwhelmed and unable to cope, or they may react by wanting to learn more about diabetes.

HUMANISTIC A way of thought or action concerned with the interests or ideals of people.

HYPOTHESIS An assertion subject to verification or proof. (Compare with *A*ssumption and *I*nference.)

IMPLY To express indirectly, to hint or suggest. To suggest by logical necessity.

INDEPENDENT NURSING ACTIONS Nursing actions performed independently, without need for physician's orders or facility protocols. For example, ensuring adequate oral intake to prevent dehydration. (Compare with *C*ollaborative actions.)

INDEPENDENT NURSING INTERVENTION See *I*ndependent nursing actions.

INDICATOR A criterion for evaluating progress toward a goal.

INDUCTIVE REASONING Drawing *general* conclusions by observing a few *specific* members of a class. For example: "Since everyone I ever knew with a bacterial infection required an antibiotic, and Jane has a bacterial infection, Jane requires an antibiotic." (Compare with *D*eductive reasoning.)

INFER To suspect something, or to attach meaning to information. For example, if someone is frowning, we may infer that he or she is worried.

INFERENCE Something we suspect to be true, based on logical conclusion after examination of evidence. (Compare with *A*ssumption and *H*ypothesis.)

INTERVENTION Something done to prevent, cure, or control a health problem (e.g., turning someone every 2 hours is an intervention to prevent skin breakdown).

INTUBATION The process of inserting a tube into an individual's bronchus in order to facilitate breathing.

INTUITION Knowing something without evidence.

IRRIGATE To flush a tube (with normal saline solution or water) to keep it *patent*.

LIFE PROCESSES Events or changes that occur during one's lifetime (e.g., growing up, getting married, losing someone).

LOGIC A system of reasoning that leads to valid conclusions.

MEASURABLE Capable of being clearly observed so that the quality or quantity of something can be determined.

MEDICAL DIAGNOSIS A problem with structure or function of an organ or system requiring definitive diagnosis and treatment by a qualified physician.

MEDICAL DOMAIN Actions a physician is legally qualified to perform.

MENTOR A knowledgeable, insightful, and trusted person who helps someone else clarify thinking.

METACOGNITION An awareness of how to think and what dispositions or behaviors improve thinking; "thinking about your thinking while you're thinking" (Pesut, 1992). Sometimes used interchangeably with *critical thinking*.

MORAL Concerned with the judgment of whether a human action or character is right or wrong.

MYOCARDIAL INFARCTION Partial or complete occlusion of one or more of the coronary arteries, causing death of coronary tissue.

NASOGASTRIC TUBE A tube inserted into through the nose, down the esophagus, and into the stomach.

NURSE-PRESCRIBED INTERVENTION An action prescribed by a nurse. For example, "Turn the patient every 2 hours."

NURSING DIAGNOSIS A clinical judgment about an individual, family, or community response to actual or potential health problems and life processes. Nursing diagnoses provide the basis for selection of nursing interventions to achieve outcomes for which the nurse is accountable (NANDA, 1990).

NURSING DOMAIN Actions a nurse is legally qualified to perform.

NURSING PROCESS The method used by nurses to expedite diagnosis and treatment of actual and potential health problems.

OBJECTIVE DATA Information that you can clearly observe or measure. For example, a pulse of 140 beats per minute.

OUTCOME The result of prescribed interventions; usually refers to the *expected result* or goal of interventions. (See also *Client-centered goal*.)

PARADIGM (pa'-ra-dīm) A way of thinking that helps us understand and improve how something is accomplished (e.g., see Paradigm Change Is Transformational on page 1).

PATENT Open, so as to allow the flow of fluid or air.

PATIENT-CENTERED GOAL See *Client-centered outcome*.

PHYSICIAN-PRESCRIBED INTERVENTION An action prescribed by a physician for other professionals to perform.

POLICIES See *Guidelines*.

POTENTIAL DIAGNOSIS A problem or diagnosis that may occur because of certain risk factors present (e.g., someone who's on prolonged bed rest has a potential for skin breakdown. (Compare with *High-risk diagnosis*.)

POTENTIAL PROBLEM See *Potential diagnosis*.

PRECEPTOR An experienced, more qualified nurse assigned by a facility to facilitate learning for a less experienced nurse.

PROACTIVE (comes from *act before*) A way of thinking and behaving that accepts responsibility for one's actions and takes initiative to plan ahead to anticipate and prevent problems before they happen.

PROCEDURES See *Guidelines*.

PROTOCOLS See *Guidelines*.

PULMONARY EMBOLUS A clot that has blocked off circulation and oxygenation to lung tissue. Considered to be life-threatening.

QA See *Quality assessment*.

QI See *Quality improvement*.

QUALIFIED Having the competence and authority to perform an action.

QUALITY The degree to which patient care services increase the probability of achieving *desired* outcomes with the decreased probability of *undesired* outcomes.

QUALITY ASSESSMENT (QA) Ongoing studies designed to evaluate quality of patient care and services. Just as *assessment* is the first step of the nursing process, QA is the first step of QI (quality improvement).

QUALITY CARE Health care services that increase the probability of achieving *desired* results with decreased probability of *undesired* results.

QUALITY IMPROVEMENT (QI) Ongoing studies designed to identify ways to promote achievement of desired outcomes in a timely, cost-effective fashion, while decreasing the risks for undesired outcomes.

RALES Abnormal breath sounds (crackles) caused by the passage of air through bronchi containing fluid. This sign is frequently associated with congestive heart failure.

RELATED FACTOR See *R*isk factor.

RESPONSE A reaction of an organism or person to a specific mechanism.

RISK FACTOR Something known to contribute to (or be associated with) a specific problem. (See also *E*tiology.)

RISK NURSING DIAGNOSIS Human response to health conditions or life processes which may develop in a vulnerable individual, family or community. Supported by risk factors that contribute to increased vulnerability (NANDA, 1994).

RULE A standard of behavior or practice that, when used as a guide, can enhance your ability to achieve your goals.

SHORT-TERM GOAL A client-centered outcome that's achieved as a stepping stone to reaching a long-term goal.

SIGNS Objective data that cause you to suspect a health problem.

SOMNOLENT Overly sleepy; difficult to arouse.

STANDARDS OF CARE See *G*uidelines.

SUBJECTIVE DATA Information the patient states or communicates; the patient's perceptions. For example, "My heart feels like it's racing."

SYMPATHY Sharing the same feelings as another. (Compare with *E*mpathy.)

SYMPTOMS Subjective data that cause you to suspect a health problem.

SYNTHESIS The process of putting pieces of information together to make a whole. For example, nurses put individual signs and symptoms together to make a diagnosis.

THROMBI More than one thrombus. (See *T*hrombus.)

THROMBUS A clot that threatens blood supply to tissues. If the clot moves, it becomes an *embolus*.

TUBAL LIGATION Surgery performed to sterilize a female by cutting and suturing the fallopian tubes.

VALIDATION The process of gathering more data to determine whether the information or data you've already collected are factual or true.

VALIDITY The extent to which something can be believed to be factual and true.

WELLNESS DIAGNOSIS A clinical judgment about an individual, family, or community in transition from a specific level of wellness to a higher level of wellness (NANDA, 1990).

Alfaro-LeFevre, R. (1994). *Applying nursing process: A step by step guide* (3rd ed.). Philadelphia: J.B. Lippincott.

Alfaro-LeFevre, R. (1994). Teaching nurses critical thinking. *Academy of Medical-Surgical News,* 3 (2), 4, 8.

American Nurses Association (1980). *A social policy statement.* Kansas City, MO: American Nurses Association.

Arnold, E., and Boggs, K. (1994) *Interpersonal relationships: Professional communication skills for nurses* (2nd ed.). Philadelphia: W.B. Saunders Co.

Barnes, C., and McCabe, N. (1992). *Critical thinking: Educational imperatives.* San Francisco: Jossey-Bass Publishers.

Becker, H. (1994). Indicators of critical thinking, communication, and therapeutic interventions among first line nursing supervisors. *Nurse Educator,* 19 (2), 15–19.

Benner, P. (1984). *From novice to expert.* Menlo Park, CA: Addison-Wesley.

Berry, R. (1993). Effective patient education, part 1: Teaching adults. *Nursing Spectrum (PA Ed),* 2 (23), 14–16.

Bevis, E. (1988). New directions for a new age. In National League for Nursing, *Curriculum revolution: Mandate for change* (pp. 27–52). New York: NLN.

Bloom, B. (Ed.) (1956). *Taxonomy of educational objectives.* Handbook 1, Cognitive domain. New York: McKay.

Bowers, B. (1993). Developing analytic thinking skills in early undergraduate education. *Journal of Nursing Education,* 32 (3), 107–114.

Brigham, C. (1993). Nursing education and critical thinking: Interplay of content and thinking. *Holistic Nurse Practice,* 7 (3), 48–54.

Brix, A. (1993). Critical thinking and theory-based practice. *Holistic Nurse Practice,* 7 (3), 21–27.

Brookfield, S. (1989). *Developing critical thinkers: Challenging adults to explore alternative ways of thinking and acting.* San Francisco: Jossey-Bass.

Brown, H. (1994) *Life's little instruction book.* Nashville: Rutledge Press.

Brown, H., and Sorrell, J. (1993). Use of clinical journals to enhance critical thinking. *Nurse Educator,* 18 (5), 16–18.

Bucher, L. (1993). The effects of imagery abilities and mental rehearsal on learning a nursing skill. *Journal of Nursing Education,* 32 (7), 318–324.

Burfitt, S., Greiner, D., and Miers, L. (1993). Professional nurse caring as perceived by critically ill patients: A phenomenologic study. *American Journal of Critical Care,* 2 (6), 489–499.

Burns, N., and Groves, S. (1993) *The practice of nursing research: Conduct, critique, and utilization* (2nd ed.). Philadelphia: W.B. Saunders Co.

Carpenito, L. (1993). *Nursing diagnosis: Application to clinical practice* (5th ed.). Philadelphia: J.B. Lippincott.

Carper, B. (1978). Fundamental patterns of knowing in nursing. *Advances in Nursing Science,* 1 (1), 13–23.

Costello, K. (1993). The Myers-Briggs type indicator— management tool. *Nursing Management,* 24 (5), 46–47, 50–51.

Covey, S. (1994). *Daily reflections for highly effective people.* New York: Simon & Schuster.

Covey, S. (1989). *The seven habits of highly effective people.* New York: Simon & Schuster. Excerpts of *The Seven Habits of Highly Effective People*® used with permission of Covey Leadership Center, Inc., 3507 N. University Ave. P.O. Box 19008, Provo, Utah, 84604-4479. Phone: (800) 331-7716.

Deering, C. (1993). Giving and taking criticism. *American Journal of Nursing,* 93 (12), 56–58.

del Bueno, D. (1990). Experience, education and nurses' ability to make clinical judgments. *Nursing and Health Care,* 11 (6), 290–294.

del Bueno, D. (1994). Guest Editorial: Why can't new grads think like nurses? *Nurse Educator,* 19 (4), 9–11.

Dickensen-Hazard, N. (1989). Making the grade as a test taker. *Pediatric Nursing,* 15, 302–304.

Dickensen-Hazard, N. (1989). Anatomy of a test question. *Pediatric Nursing,* 15, 480–481.

Dickensen-Hazard, N. (1990). The psychology of successful test taking. *Pediatric Nursing,* 16, 66–67.

Dracup, K., and Bryan-Brown, C. (1994). The three R's: Reading, writing, and research. *American Journal of Critical Care,* 3 (5), 329–330.

Ennis, R. (1987). A taxonomy of critical thinking dispositions and abilities. In J.B. Baron and J.J. Sternberg (eds.), *Teaching thinking skills: Theory and practice.* New York: Freeman.

Ennis, R. (1990). Experience, education, and nurses' ability to make clinical judgments. *Nursing and Health Care,* 11 (6), 290–294.

Facione, P. (1990). *Critical thinking: A statement of expert consensus for purposes of education assessment and instruction.* Research findings and recommendations prepared for the Committee on Pre-College Philosophy of the American Psychological Association.

Ferguson, M. (1980). *Aquarian conspiracy: Personal and social transformation in our time.* New York: G.P. Putnam's Sons.

Fishman, M., Hoffman, A., Klaus, R., and Thaler, M. (1991). *Medicine* (p. v). Philadelphia: J.B. Lippincott.

Fonteyn, M. (1991). Implications of clinical reasoning studies for critical care nursing. *Focus,* 18 (4), 322–327.

Foster, P. (1993). Helping students learn to make ethical decisions. *Holistic Nurse Practice,* 7 (3), 28–35.

Gardner, H. (1993) *Multiple intelligences.* New York: Basic Books.

Gordon, M. (1987). *Nursing diagnosis: Process and application.* New York: McGraw-Hill.

Gruca, J. (1994). Bug of the week: A personification teaching strategy. *Journal of Nursing Education,* 33 (4), 153–154.

Halpern, D. (1984). *Thought and knowledge.* Hillsdale, NJ: Lawrence Erlbaum Associates.

Hartman, D. (1993). Critical thinking in psychiatric nursing in the decade of the brain. *Holistic Nurse Practice,* 7 (3), 55–63.

Iyer, P., Taptich, B., and Bernnochi-Losey, D. (1991). *Nursing process and nursing diagnosis* (2nd ed.). Philadelphia: W.B. Saunders Co.

Jameton, A. (1984). *Nursing practice: The ethical issues.* Englewood Cliffs, NJ: Prentice-Hall.

Jeffries, M. (1993). Guided visual metaphor: A creative strategy for teaching nursing diagnosis. *Nursing Diagnosis,* 4 (3), 99–106.

Jenks, J. (1993). The pattern of personal knowing in nurse clinical decision making. *Journal of Nursing Education,* 32 (9), 399–405.

Jones, S., and Brown, L. (1993). Alternative view on defining critical thinking through the nursing process. *Holistic Nurse Practice,* 7 (3), 71–76.

Kamii, C. (1991). Toward autonomy: The importance of critical thinking and choice making. *School Psychology Review,* 20 (3), 382–388.

Keane, M. (1993). Preferred learning styles and study strategies in a linguistically diverse baccalaureate nursing student population. *Journal of Nursing Education,* 32 (5), 215–221.

Kemper, B. (1992). Therapeutic listening: Developing the concept. *Journal of Psychosocial Nursing,* 29 (9), 11–15.

Kintgen-Andrews, J. (1991). Critical thinking and nursing education: Perplexities and insights. *Journal of Nursing Education,* 30 (4), 152–157.

Klaassens, E. (1988). Improving teaching for thinking. *Nurse Educator,* 13 (6), 15–19.

Kolb, D (1976). *Learning style inventory: Self-scoring test and interpretation booklet.* Boston: McBer & Co.

Komelasky, A., and Bond, B. (1993). The effect of two forms of learning reinforcement upon parental retention of CPR skills. *Pediatric Nursing,* 19 (1), 77, 96–98.

Kramer, M. (1993). Concept clarification and critical thinking: Integrated processes. *Journal of Nursing Education,* 32 (9), 387.

Kurfiss, J. (1988). *Critical thinking: Theory, research, practice, and possibilities.* ASHE-ERIC Higher Education Report No. 2. Washington, DC: Association for the Study of Higher Education.

Lashley, M., and Wittstadt, R. (1993). Writing across the curriculum: An integrated curricular approach to developing critical thinking through writing. *Journal of Nursing Education,* 32 (9), 422–424.

Loving, G. (1993). Competence validation and cognitive flexibility: A theoretical mode grounded in nursing education. *Journal of Nursing Education,* 32 (9), 387.

McPeck, J. (1981). *Critical thinking and education.* New York: St Martin's.

McKenzie, L. (1992). Critical thinking in healthcare supervision. *Health Care Supervisor,* 10 (4), 1–11.

Meyers, C. (1986). *Teaching students to think critically.* San Francisco: Jossey-Bass.

Meyers, I. B. (1987). *Introduction to type: A description of the theory and applications of the Meyers-Briggs type indicator.* Palo Alto, CA: Consulting Psychologists Press.

Miller, M., and Malcolm, N. (1990). Critical thinking in the nursing curriculum. *Nursing and Health Care,* 11 (2), 67–73.

Mollan-Masters, R. (1992). *You are smarter than you think.* Ashland, OR: Reality Productions.

National League for Nursing (1989). *Role and competencies of graduates of diploma programs in nursing.* New York: NLN.

National League for Nursing (1990). *Educational outcomes of associate degree nursing programs: Roles and competencies.* New York: NLN.

National League for Nursing (1991). *Criteria for the evaluation of baccalaureate and higher degree programs in nursing* (6th ed.). New York: NLN.

Norman, G. (1988). Problem-solving skills, solving problems, and problem-based learning. *Medical Education,* 22, 279–286.

North American Nursing Diagnosis Association (1990). *Taxonomy I* (rev. ed.). St. Louis, MO: NANDA.

North American Nursing Diagnosis Association (1994). *NANDA guidelines for nursing diagnosis submission.* Philadelphia: NANDA.

Ouellette, F. (1988). A textbook coding tool: Part 1, Assessing elements that promote analytic abilities. *Nurse Educator,* 13 (5), 8–13.

Parish, A. (1994). It only hurts when I don't laugh. *American Journal of Nursing,* 94 (8), 47.

Paul, R. (1992). Critical thinking: What, why, and how? In C. Barnes (ed.), *Critical thinking, an educational imperative.* San Fransisco: Jossey-Bass Publishers.

Paul, R. (1993). *Critical thinking: How to prepare students for a rapidly changing world.* Santa Rosa, CA: Foundation for Critical Thinking.

Paul, R., and Binker, A. (eds.) (1990). *Critical thinking: What every person needs to survive in a rapidly changing world.* Rohner Park, CA: Foundation for Critical Thinking and Moral Development.

Pesut, D., and Herman, J. (1992). Metacognitive skills in diagnostic reasoning: Making the implicit explicit. *Nursing Diagnosis,* 3 (4), 148–153.

Pless, B., and Clayton, G. (1993). Clarifying the concept of critical thinking in nursing. *Journal of Nursing Education,* 32 (9), 387.

Pond, E., Bradshaw, M., and Turner, S. (1991). Teaching strategies for clinical thinking. *Nurse Educator,* 16 (6), 18–22.

Reilly, D. (Ed.) (1978). *Teaching and evaluating the affective domain in nursing programs.* Thorofare, NJ: Charles B. Slack.

Rittman, M., Nedonma, N., Quesenberry, L., et al. (1993). Learning from "never again" stories. *American Journal of Nursing,* 93 (6), 40–43.

Robinson, A. (1993). *What smart students know: Maximum grades, optimum learning, minimum time.* New York: Crown Trade Paperbacks.

Ruggiero, V. (1988). *Teaching thinking across the curriculum.* New York: Harper & Row.

Ruggiero, V. (1991). *The art of thinking: A guide to critical and creative thought* (3rd ed). New York: HarperCollins.

Saarmann, L., Freitas, L., Rapps, J., and Riegel, B. (1992). The relationship of education to critical thinking ability and values among nurses: Socialization into professional nursing. *Journal of Professional Nursing,* 8 (1), 26–34.

Schoessler, M., Conedera, F., Bell, L., et al. (1993). Use of the Myers-Briggs type indicator to develop a continuing education department. *Journal of Nursing Staff Development,* 9 (1), 8–13.

Sides, M., and Korchek, N. (1994). *Nurses guide to successful test-taking* (2nd ed.). Philadelphia: J.B. Lippincott.

Tanner, C. (1983). Research on clinical judgment. In W.L. Holzemer (ed.), *Review of Research in Nursing Education* (pp. 1–32). Thorofare, NJ: Charles B. Slack.

Tanner, C. (1993a). More about critical thinking and clinical decision making. *Journal of Nursing Education,* 32 (9), 387.

Tanner, C. (1993b). Thinking about critical thinking. *Journal of Nursing Education,* 32(9), 99–100.

Tanner, C., Benner, P., Chesla, C., and Gordon, D. (1993) The phenomenology of knowing the patient. *Image,* 25 (4), 273–280.

Taylor, C., Lillis, C., and Lamone, P. (1993). *Fundamentals of Nursing: The art and science of nursing care* (2nd ed.). Philadelphia: J.B. Lippincott.

Tschikota, S. (1993). The clinical decision-making processes of student nurses. *Journal of Nursing Education,* 32 (9), 387.

Valiga, T. (1983). Cognitive development: A critical component of baccalaureate nursing education. *Image,* 15, 115–119.

Von Oech, R. (1983). *A whack on the side of the head: How you can be more creative.* New York: Warner Books.

Watson, G., and Glaser, E. (1964). *Critical thinking appraisal manual.* New York, New York: Harcourt, Brace, & World.

Worrell, P. (1990). Metacognition: Implication for instruction in nursing education. *Journal of Nursing Education,* 29 (4).

Index